DATE DUE

GAYLORD			PRINTED IN U.S.A.

Digital Medicine

Digital Medicine
HEALTH CARE IN THE INTERNET ERA

Darrell M. West
Edward Alan Miller

BROOKINGS INSTITUTION PRESS
Washington, D.C.

Copyright © 2009
THE BROOKINGS INSTITUTION
1775 Massachusetts Avenue, N.W., Washington, D.C. 20036
www.brookings.edu

Library of Congress Cataloging-in-Publication data
West, Darrell M., 1954–
  Digital medicine : health care in the Internet era / Darrell M. West, Edward Alan Miller.
      p. ;   cm.
  Includes bibliographical references and index.
  Summary: "Investigates factors limiting the ability of digital technology to remake health care. Analyzes data sources to study content of health care-related websites, sponsorship status, public usage, and the relationship between e-health use and health care attitudes. Examines the different ways in which officials overseas have implemented health information technology"—Provided by publisher.
  ISBN 978-0-8157-0276-4 (cloth : alk. paper)
  1. Internet in medicine. 2. Medical informatics. I. Miller, Edward Alan. II. Brookings Institution. III. Title.
  [DNLM: 1. Medical Informatics. 2. Internet. 3. Telemedicine. W 26.5 W517d 2009]
  R859.7.I58W47 2009
  610.285'46—dc22   2009006454

1 3 5 7 9 8 6 4 2

Printed on acid-free paper

Typeset in Sabon with Myriad display

Composition by Cynthia Stock
Silver Spring, Maryland

Printed by R. R. Donnelley
Harrisonburg, Virginia

To the memory of Bob and Jean West

and to

Edward Miller's mother, Diane Miller Asche;

late father, Allen Miller;

and late stepfather, Edwin Asche.

Contents

Appendixes

Preface

Information technology affects virtually every aspect of human existence. People use the Internet for commerce and entertainment. They buy books, movies, and games online. Governments allow citizens to file tax returns and vehicle registration renewals digitally. In many jurisdictions, people pay fees electronically or register complaints about potholes, rats, and garbage collection through designated websites.

With the explosion of online activity, policy advocates hope to bring the benefits of information technology to health care. Governments, hospitals, doctors, and pharmaceutical manufacturers have placed a tremendous amount of medical information online in recent years. Rather than personally visit or call health care professionals, patients can surf websites filled with detailed information about specific illnesses, order drugs and equipment online, and communicate with physicians or other health professionals through e-mail or web messaging. Advances in information technology give people more powerful communications choices than at any other point in human history.

However, there are a variety of political, social, ethical, and economic forces that limit the scope of the electronic health revolution. Medical care is a highly politicized policy area characterized by intense conflict between major interests. Responsibility for health care is shared among fragmented financing and service delivery systems, which slows the pace of change. Reform is complicated by a digital divide that prevents many vulnerable populations from taking full advantage of recent advances in information technology. Technology costs, ethical dilemmas, and privacy concerns make it difficult for society to take full advantage of new modes of communication within the health care sphere.

This book investigates factors that limit the ability of digital technology to remake health care. Few people use the Internet to search for health information, purchase prescription drugs online, or e-mail health care providers. Most do not avail themselves of electronic medical records. Based on our analysis of online content, national public opinion surveys, and case studies of technology innovation, we argue that gains in health information technology will not be realized until policymakers and health care officials develop a better understanding of key problems. A variety of measures are required to bring health information technology to all consumers. Prevailing obstacles in the form of political divisions, technology costs, communications problems, ethical issues, privacy concerns, and disparities between social groups must be addressed if the benefits of the e-health revolution are to be extended to all.

Chapter 1 of this volume takes stock of the revolution in health information technology that has unfolded in recent years. From websites featuring the latest on diseases and drugs to electronic medical records and digital communications with health care professionals, patients have a range of options for supplementing conventional face-to-face and telephone interactions: e-mail, website visits, online purchases, and storage of medical information in electronic form. We review the rise of e-health in health care and the benefits in quality, accessibility, and affordability that proponents hope to gain through more widespread use of advanced communications technology. We argue that a variety of factors have limited use and that those obstacles must be overcome if the e-health revolution is to reach its full potential.

Chapter 2 compares health care material on government websites to that found in the private and nonprofit sectors. Using a content analysis of health sites, we find that private websites are more likely to display potential conflicts of interest because they accept advertising from interested parties and are sponsored by for-profit organizations. Those factors pose serious problems for consumers needing accurate, comprehensive, and unbiased information. In addition, private sites are more likely to follow "niche" strategies, which target particular groups of people based on age, gender, race, income, or specific disease. Rather than providing material of interest to a wide range of consumers, these sites differentiate based on market segments. Taken together, these concerns limit the scope of the e-health revolution and make it difficult to achieve the service improvements and cost savings envisioned by policy advocates.

Chapter 3 examines the extent to which people actually use information technology for health care. Relative to face-to-face and telephone interactions, how many people e-mail health care providers, visit webpages for medical information, and order prescription drugs or medical equipment online? Drawing on a national survey that we conducted, we find that relatively few Americans make use of health information technology and that a variety of barriers limit people's usage of digital health resources. Low use rates pose serious problems for the future of electronic health.

Chapter 4 looks at the relationship between health information technology and attitudes toward health care affordability, quality, and accessibility. In our national survey, we find that health information technology users are no more likely to have positive views about quality, access, and affordability than individuals who rely on personal or telephone interactions with health care providers. Those findings suggest that e-health utilization is not producing attitude or perception shifts of the sort desired by policy advocates.

One of the most pressing problems in health care is inequitable quality and access, including differences by age, race, gender, income, education, and geography. Unfortunately, many of the very same disparities have carried over and been reinforced by the recent growth of the health care Internet. Chapter 5 investigates whether the factors influencing visits to health websites vary by various demographic characteristics. We find that Hispanics with low literacy are less likely than other social groups to visit health websites. Prevailing disparities of this sort limit the ability of health information technology to help large segments of consumers and seriously constrain the overall effectiveness of the e-health revolution in improving U.S. health care.

Chapter 6 analyzes visits to public and private health care websites. We find that people are more than twice as likely to visit private as public sector websites, in part because of the greater marketing efforts of commercial enterprises. We document differences in the characteristics of those seeking medical information from these alternative sources of information. Younger individuals who live in urban areas and who have stronger health literacy and report greater concerns about health care affordability are more likely to visit privately sponsored but not publicly sponsored websites. Those findings imply that efforts to close the digital divide must recognize differences in user characteristics across government and non-government website providers in order to be effective.

In chapter 7, we go beyond the U.S. experience and look at health information technology innovation around the world. Adoption of electronic health records by primary care physicians in the United States has lagged behind adoption in countries such as the United Kingdom. Furthermore, other countries have invested far more than the United States in health information technology, including development of high-quality, interoperable systems that enable providers from different regions to communicate with one another. They include many Asian and European countries that have devoted considerable resources to making broadband technology widely available, thereby accelerating their use of health information technology. To better understand these developments, we present the results of successful innovation in other nations and compare the national government health websites of countries around the world.

In chapter 8, we focus on ways to reduce disparities in use of health information technology. We examine a number of different approaches, such as boosting literacy in regard to health information technology, providing low-cost technology (that is, laptops or personal digital assistants), training medical professionals, overcoming legal and political obstacles, and taking ethics and privacy seriously. We argue that technology in and of itself will not improve health care unless consumers and health professionals obtain further training and better equipment that lowers extant barriers. While it still is early in the technology revolution, this book suggests that with specific adjustments and improved training, health information technology can boost usage and thereby transform service delivery and citizen attitudes about health care. The key is for policymakers to adopt strategies that will reap the maximum benefits of the information revolution in health care.

We are grateful to many organizations and individuals for their assistance on this project. The Taubman Center for Public Policy at Brown University provided financial support for our research, and the John Hazen White Public Opinion Laboratory made possible the national survey undertaken for this book. The Taubman Center and the Governance Studies program at the Brookings Institution provided a hospitable home for writing the final chapters. Marykate Bergen did great work as a research assistant on this project. She collected data, compiled background information, and edited the manuscript. We are very grateful for her many contributions to our book. We would like to thank Bob Faherty, Chris Kelaher, Mary Kwak, Eileen Hughes, and Susan Woollen of Brookings Press for their speedy and professional handling of the manuscript. None of these individuals or organizations, however, bears any responsibility for the arguments we make in this volume.

Digital Medicine

CHAPTER ONE

The E-Health Revolution

Websites such as WebMD.com, MedlinePlus.gov, MerckSource.com, HealthFinder.gov, and MayoClinic.com answer health-related questions and provide links to discussion groups about particular illnesses. In states such as Massachusetts, California, New York, and Michigan, consumers can visit state health department sites and compare performance data on the quality of care. The U.S. government has a website that evaluates 2,500 hospitals on mortality rates, room cleanliness, and call button response and on how their patients judge the quality of the care that they provide.[1] Some physicians encourage patients to use e-mail or web messaging instead of telephone calls or in-office visits for simple issues such as appointments, prescription renewals, referrals, or brief consultations. And digital diagnostic systems, decision-support software for health care providers, telemedicine (medical care provided by televideo or telephone), and computer-aided self-help tools also are available.

Despite the wealth of digital medicine applications available through e-mail, the Internet, and mobile devices, not many physicians or patients are taking advantage of the potential of electronic communications. Only 15 percent of the 560,000 doctors in the United States use the Internet to order medication for their patients.[2] Industry advocates claim that a move to electronic prescriptions could save $29 billion over the next decade. According to health experts, digital technology would save money and "make transactions more efficient, reduce medication errors, and entice doctors to prescribe less expensive drugs."[3]

Some observers, however, worry that these types of electronic consultations will depersonalize health care. Social medicine expert Helen Hughes Evans, for example, argues that "technology has stripped medicine of its humanistic qualities" and that doctors rely too heavily on high-tech instruments.[4] She feels that rather than advancing the quality of patient care, digital medicine has undermined the intimacy of clinician-patient relations among those who rely on electronic devices and therefore has contributed to the loss of the personal touch in the provision of health care.

In a review of research on telemedicine, though, Edward Alan Miller finds that 80 percent of medical studies showed a favorable impact of digitally mediated contact on provider-patient relations.[5] Digital technologies facilitate access to health care for some individuals and expand the network of available health care providers. Digital communications allow people with rare diseases to find others who suffer from the same disorders and to learn from their experiences. Moreover, digital systems allow patients to take advantage of specialists in other states and even other countries. Although technology often appears to be "dehumanizing," studies suggest that it can increase resources for self-care, enhance emotional support through electronic support groups, and improve knowledge regarding special medical problems.

In this book, we examine the revolution in information technology that is taking place in health care, the presumed benefits of electronic or digital health care, and barriers to technological innovation. We argue that in order to achieve the promise of health information technology, digital medicine must overcome the barriers created by political divisions, fragmented jurisdiction, the digital divide, the cost of technology, ethical conflicts, and privacy concerns. The desired cost savings and service improvements in health care cannot be achieved without addressing those matters.[6]

USE OF ONLINE INFORMATION

Since the mid-1990s, there has been a dramatic increase in overall Internet use in the United States. According to figures compiled by the Pew Internet and American Life Project, 73 percent of respondents in 2006 said that they used the Internet, up from 14 percent in 1995. As shown in figure 1-1, Internet usage in the United States has risen steadily in

FIGURE 1-1. Internet Usage in the United States

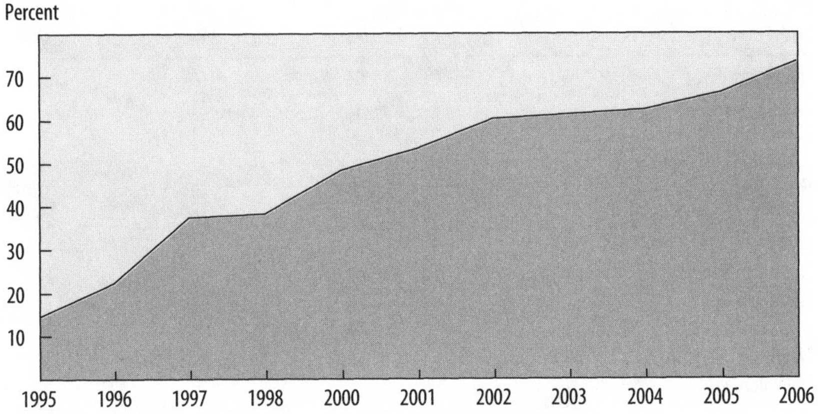

Percent

Source: Pew Internet and American Life Project National Surveys, 2002, 2004, and 2006.

recent years. In 2006, 66 percent of respondents said that they were Internet users, indicating a 7 percentage-point gain from 2005 to 2006.

Patients face a dizzying variety of new ways to communicate with medical providers and gain information about health care problems.[7] They can search websites devoted to medical ailments, e-mail health care professionals, buy medicines and health care products online, and engage in interactive communication with medical providers. Such options offer people more control over their health care while also improving the quality and affordability of treatments.[8]

However, few Americans are taking advantage of health information technologies. In a Wall Street Journal Online/Harris Interactive Health-Care Poll of 2,624 adults across the nation, only a small number of respondents indicated that they used electronic technologies to communicate with health care providers. Four percent got reminders through e-mail from their doctor when they were due for a visit, 4 percent used e-mail to communicate directly with their doctor, 3 percent scheduled appointments through the Internet, 2 percent received the results of diagnostic tests through e-mail, 2 percent had access to electronic medical records, and 2 percent relied on home monitoring devices that allowed them to e-mail blood pressure readings directly to their doctor's office.[9]

When asked whether they would like to employ such technologies, large majorities indicated that they would do so if they had the opportunity. The survey shows that respondents would like the following options:

TABLE 1-1. Health Topics Searched for Online by Internet Users
Percent of users

Health topic	2002	2004	2006
Specific disease	63	66	64
Certain medical treatment	47	51	51
Diet or nutrition	44	51	49
Exercise	36	42	44
Medical drugs	34	40	37
Particular doctor or hospital	21	28	29
Health insurance	25	31	28
Alternative treatments	28	30	27
Mental health	21	23	22
Environmental health	17	18	22
Experimental treatments	18	23	18
Immunizations	13	16	16
Dental health	—	—	15
Medicare/Medicaid	9	11	13
Sexual health	10	11	11
Quitting smoking	6	7	9
Drug/alcohol problems	8	8	8

Source: Pew Internet and American Life Project National Surveys, 2002, 2004, and 2006.

—to get an e-mail reminder when they are due for an appointment (77 percent)

—to use e-mail to communicate directly with their doctor (74 percent)

—to receive the results of diagnostic tests through e-mail (67 percent)

—to schedule an appointment through the Internet (75 percent)

—to have an electronic medical record (64 percent)

—to use a home monitoring device that allows them to e-mail blood pressure readings to their doctor's office (57 percent).[10]

Those who went online for medical information most commonly searched for information on specific diseases. As shown in table 1-1, of those who went online, 64 percent said that they searched for information on particular illnesses, 51 percent for information on certain medical treatments, 49 percent for information on diet and nutrition, and 44 percent for information on exercise; 37 percent sought advice on medical drugs, and 29 percent looked for particular doctors or hospitals. The number of people searching online for medical information increased in most categories during the 2002–06 period covered by the surveys.

Of those who went online for health or medical information, 58 percent indicated that the information affected their health care decisions,

55 percent said that it changed their approach to health care, and 54 percent reported that it prompted them to ask new questions of their medical providers. When asked how the information made them feel, 74 percent said that they felt reassured and 56 percent felt more confident, but 25 percent indicated that they were overwhelmed by the amount of online information, 18 percent were confused by the information, and 10 percent were frightened by information.[11]

From those findings, it is clear that some people have positive experiences that help them learn more about illnesses and treatments but that others have difficulty dealing with the new world of online information. They do not feel comfortable searching for information online, and they get confused or overwhelmed by what they find at medical websites. Although the positive views outweigh the negative, significant segments of the population still feel queasy about employing digital medicine to meet their own health care needs.

BENEFITS OF ELECTRONIC HEALTH

Concerns about health care quality, affordability, and accessibility have led policymakers in recent years to see more widespread adoption of health information technology as a way to improve the efficiency and effectiveness of health care and to cut costs. Through Internet websites, broadband access, e-mail communications, online procurement, and electronic record keeping, national leaders see digital technology as a valuable tool for bringing U.S. health care into the twenty-first century.[12]

The United States spends $2 trillion a year on health care, which is around 16 percent of the gross domestic product.[13] That is twice the amount spent in 1995, when spending topped $1 trillion for the first time. With health care spending increasing at 6.7 percent a year, expenditures are projected to rise to 20 percent of GDP by 2015.[14] Medicaid spending has increased by more than 45 percent, to $311 billion, since 2000. Medicare spending has risen by 38 percent and now exceeds $400 billion.[15] Health insurance premiums have shown double-digit increases in recent years, well above the rate of inflation.[16]

Rising costs have placed enormous pressures on public and private health care systems. Although individual consumers typically report a high level of satisfaction with their personal care, the United States performs poorly on a variety of aggregate health indicators.[17] Forty-five million

Americans (about 17 percent) lack access to health insurance.[18] U.S. life expectancy trails that of other industrialized countries.[19]

In such circumstances, many people worry whether they are receiving adequate care and treatment, especially in light of widespread reporting of adverse drug events and other problems.[20] Around 98,000 Americans die each year because of medical errors.[21] Others distrust managed care and the incentives it offers health providers to control costs by restricting treatment.[22]

To deal with competing demands for economy, efficiency, and effectiveness, expenditures on health information technology are rising rapidly. In 2000, the United States spent around $19 billion in this area; according to the American Hospital Association, the figure jumped to $31 billion in 2006. The typical health care organization devotes a modest 2.5 percent of its annual budget to information technology, about the same as public sector organizations in other policy areas.[23] Much of that investment is designed to deliver services while keeping expenses at reasonable levels.

In 2004, President George W. Bush signed an executive order creating the Office of the National Coordinator for Health Information Technology, which is charged with devising medical policies that use technology to improve health care quality, reduce costs, and coordinate medical care among different medical professionals. The goal is to use new technologies to facilitate a variety of functions, including diagnostic support, computerized physician order entry and verification, electronic claims processing and eligibility checking, secure communications, alternative information gathering, and electronic reminders.

Former U.S. House Speaker Newt Gingrich sees information technology as a panacea for service problems and rising health care costs.[24] Gingrich believes that patients can be empowered and errors in patient records reduced through electronic medical records and digital communications with doctors. Rather than allowing medical costs to continue to spiral out of control, health care professionals can use these new tools to cut costs while giving consumers more control over health care information.

During her presidential campaign, Senator Hillary Clinton placed health information technology at the center of her American Health Choices Plan, which called for universal coverage that would cost around $110 billion to implement. Half of the money to finance coverage would come from "public savings generated from Senator Clinton's broader agenda to modernize the health systems and reduce wasteful health spending." The savings would include money recouped from the use of electronic health records and other forms of digital medical accounting systems.[25]

In 2008, then senator Barack Obama argued that electronic technology could improve health care quality, affordability, and efficiency. He proposed investing $10 billion annually over the next five years "to move the U.S. health care system to broad adoption of standards-based electronic health information systems, including electronic health records." Obama claimed that if the nation committed sufficient funds, it would save up to $77 billion each year "through improvements such as reduced hospital stays, avoidance of duplicative and unnecessary testing, more appropriate drug utilization, and other efficiencies."[26]

Medical experts estimate that effective implementation of electronic medical records could save $81 billion a year by improving health care efficiency and safety. Financial savings could grow to twice that amount by facilitating the prevention and management of chronic disease through health information technology.[27] A study of eighty controlled clinical trials to evaluate the efficacy of distance-technology supplements to conventional clinical practice found a strong association between positive health outcomes and use of computerized and telephone communications for follow-up, counseling, reminders, screening, after-hours access, and touch-tone interactive systems. Sixty-three percent of the studies reviewed found improved performance or other significant benefits.[28]

In a separate randomized controlled trial, patients using an Internet portal through which they could send secure messages directly to their physicians as well as request appointments, prescription refills, and referrals demonstrated increased satisfaction with communication, convenience, and overall care.[29] Another study of national health care quality indicators found that adoption of health information technology reduced medication errors and improved productivity.[30] Such results suggest that health information technology offers great hope for the future to individual consumers.

Some parts of the U.S. health care system, notably Veterans Administration (VA) hospitals, already have embraced digital technology. Whereas only 15 percent of U.S. physicians employ computer order entry, 94 percent of veterans' outpatient prescriptions are ordered electronically, as are nearly all inpatient medications. A comparison of VA and non-VA facilities in twelve communities found that VA patient care "scored higher on care quality, chronic disease care, and preventive care."[31]

Ordinary Americans believe that health information technology will improve medical care. In a 2006 Wall Street Journal Online/Harris Interactive Health-Care Poll, 68 percent of those polled in a national study indicated that the use of electronic medical records would improve the quality of care that patients receive by reducing the number of redundant or unnecessary tests and procedures; 60 percent thought that electronic medical records could significantly reduce health care costs; and 55 percent believed that such records could significantly decrease the frequency of medical errors.[32] Those figures demonstrate that the potential for improvements in health care treatment through digital medicine is quite high.

BARRIERS TO INNOVATION IN TECHNOLOGY

Technology offers great hope for the future, but a number of barriers remain to successful implementation in the health care arena. The real problem in health care is not technology per se but political, social, and economic challenges that complicate the adoption of digital technologies. Ordinary people have been slow to embrace technology in managing their personal health care. Consumers worry about the confidentiality of medical records, and professionals fear that the costs of technology will outweigh the benefits.

Research suggests that patients worry that the emergence of digital medicine will lower health care quality and lead to unmet health care needs. Work by Sciamanna and colleagues, for example, suggests that patients like to be able to schedule appointments online but worry about the quality of care provided online; some patients in primary care practices were concerned, for example, that they would not receive all the tests and treatments that they might require if they relied on Internet consultations.[33]

Such obstacles have made it very difficult to gain the benefits of health information technology for the system as a whole. Individual applications often sound very promising at first. Consumers like the convenience and efficiency of digital medical resources, but unless patients, insurers, health care professionals, and public officials are able to overcome the major barriers, the electronic revolution in health care will be quite limited. As discussed below, a variety of factors have slowed the adoption of health information technology in the United States.

Political Divisions

Health care is a highly politicized policy issue that has aroused intense conflict between the major political parties and among powerful interest groups, ordinary consumers, hospitals, insurers, pharmaceutical companies, and the different levels of government. Change is difficult because most of the major actors are suspicious of the motives and aims of their adversaries. Given the intense partisanship and divisive conflict surrounding health care, it is difficult for technology advocates to convince policymakers, health officials, or ordinary folks to incorporate new information technologies into service delivery.

President Bill Clinton attempted to reform the U.S. health care system in 1993–94 but failed to get Congress to take even a single vote on his plan. Although Democrats held the presidency, Senate, and House, they were unable to reach consensus on key aspects of a new system. Opponents successfully attacked the proposal as "big government" and "inefficient bureaucracy." Support for the proposed plan for health care reform started out strong but faded over time as people learned more about it.[34]

Historically, the United States has adopted major changes in health care only about once every generation. The political divisions are so severe that, short of a crisis, it is hard to build a coalition for change. People may be dissatisfied with specific aspects of health care, but it is difficult to mobilize individuals with diverse sources of dissatisfaction into a winning coalition. The widespread polarization around this issue keeps most leaders from attempting fundamental reform or succeeding if they seek to make meaningful change. Even with costs continuing to rise and millions of Americans uninsured, political leaders remain immobilized on this key issue.

Fragmented Jurisdiction

Reform has been complicated further by the fractured responsibility for the nation's health care system and telecommunications infrastructure that exists among the different levels of government. Jurisdictional uncertainties have contributed to limited investment in health information technology by both the federal and state governments. The United States lags far behind such countries as the United Kingdom, Germany, and Canada in speed and use of broadband capabilities.[35] As "laboratories of democracy," states have long been innovators in health policy;[36]

however, different regulatory environments and interstate inequities in health care make it difficult to rationalize government efforts to coordinate technology development and implementation.[37] That is one reason why countries with more centralized health care systems have proven far more successful than the United States in adopting uniform health information standards.

Indeed, the problem of communication between incompatible digital systems is a major challenge in a decentralized system. Dubbed "interoperability," this issue is aggravated in the United States because different government jurisdictions have different legal requirements and health care providers often employ hardware and software systems that are incompatible with those of other providers. The lack of uniform technical standards across the country makes it difficult to move forward with health information technology. In centralized and hierarchical systems, authorities can mandate common technologies for health care providers. But in the United States, it has been difficult to produce agreement regarding how digital medicine should unfold. Sometimes care seems to be provided within a tower of Babel. Every locality and every hospital has a different computer operating system and none is able to connect well with others. The result has been low use of information technology. No one wants to be stuck with the equivalent of a Betamax recording system at a time when the world has moved toward other formats.

Digital Divide

Not all Americans share in the advantages of technology. National estimates indicate that between 31 and 40 percent of adults use the Internet to search for health information, 5 percent use the Internet to purchase prescription drugs online, and 5 percent use e-mail to contact health care providers.[38] Taken together, those findings indicate that the online revolution is taking place at a slower rate than hoped for by policymakers.

Researchers convened by the American Medical Informatics Association have found that "a digital divide remains for vulnerable populations most likely to be underserved."[39] There are well-documented gaps in health care in the United States, and many of the disparities have carried over into the world of digital medicine.[40] Individuals who have low incomes, who are poorly educated, and who live in rural areas have less access to quality medical care than those who have higher incomes and education and live in metropolitan communities.

One reason is that members of underserved groups are less likely to use the Internet, visit health care websites, or have broadband capability.[41] Rather than overcoming inequality, technology reinforces existing systemic inequities based on age, gender, race, income, education, and geographic location. Indeed, preliminary results indicate that poor, older, rural males who are poorly educated make less use of digital communications. Such lack of access and use limits the ability of health information technology to make a positive difference in people's lives.[42]

In addition, access to technology's benefits is limited because most online health information is written at a reading level that is well above that of many users or because it is inaccurate, incomplete, or inconsistent.[43] Higher reading levels reinforce disparities in use because, according to the most recent national statistics, literacy levels differ by income, education, race, and ethnicity.[44]

Those disparities are especially salient because of the clear links between poor health literacy and inadequate understanding of medical treatment.[45] Although barriers to adoption may be especially difficult to overcome in regions that lack the infrastructure and resources necessary to sustain health information technology use and development, the promise of e-health for improving access to health information and services should be available to everyone.[46]

The extent of the disparities also is important because of its direct relationship to service delivery and costs. Use of health information technology must increase much more if the full potential of digital medicine is to be realized. It is impossible to obtain economies of scale unless the use rate is high enough to spread the costs of technology over a wide population. Unless policymakers can overcome the gaps based on race, gender, age, education, income, and geography, it will prove difficult to achieve the gains promised by information technology proponents.[47]

Cost of Technology

The high cost of electronic technologies has slowed the digital revolution. Not only is there concern about the overall cost of new devices, there is anxiety among doctors, patients, hospitals, and insurers over who will pay. The national cost of adopting electronic health records in the United States is estimated at between $276 and $320 billion over a ten-year period. For a medium-size hospital, such a system would cost about $2.7 million in development expenses and $250,000 a year in maintenance.[48]

The overall cost of a national health information system is thought to be around $156 billion in capital investment over five years and $48 billion in annual operating expenses. About two-thirds of the investment would cover system development, while one-third would go toward making systems interoperable. For medical organizations with limited financial resources, the costs are high enough to be considered prohibitive. The result in many health facilities has been failure to invest in information technology.[49]

The major barrier to investment has been that costs are concentrated while benefits are spread out among many people, which makes it difficult to build the political coalition necessary for financing major expenditures. It is easier to delay spending due to high costs, and it is difficult for hospitals, doctors, and other medical providers who would receive funding to convince others that such funding is an effective use of public monies.

Network-based health care suffers from a problem similar to that which plagued the early days of telephony. It is hard for providers to reap the true benefits of innovation until others join the digital revolution. Just as owning a telephone offered few benefits until the owner's friends and family members also had a phone, health care providers cannot achieve all the service enhancements and cost savings of technology unless others join the network. Patients whose doctors cannot access digital records will not benefit even if the most modern systems are implemented.

Congress passed legislation in 2006 that authorized a mere $125 million in expenditures for health information technology in 2006 and $155 million in 2007. It has been estimated that the country needs to invest billions in capital and operating funds to create an adequate system, and these paltry sums show the inadequacy of proposed federal spending.[50] Much more in the way of financing needs to be invested for an industry that comprises such a substantial part of the nation's GDP.

Of the member countries of the Organization for Economic Cooperation and Development, the United States spends the most on health care but lags behind the others in adoption of health-related technology.[51] It also is behind much of the developed world in adoption of electronic medical records. According to a survey undertaken by the Office of the National Coordinator for Health Information Technology, only 10 percent of physicians use a "fully operational" device that collects and stores patients' records.[52]

Financial costs are one of the major barriers to adoption. Dick Gibson, the chief medical information officer of Providence Health System, said that adoption "is not a financial play for them right now. Most docs who do it say they do it because it's the right thing to do. We know that the patient gets most of the benefit, the health plans get the rest, and the doctor is the one who has to pay for it."[53] Gibson's remarks suggest that is is not financially viable for health care providers to invest in new technology.

Ethical Conflicts

Innovation in technology also is constrained by real or perceived conflicts of interest. Although there have been few systematic studies of the quality or accuracy of viewpoints represented, private sites are much more likely to feature product ads and to push products manufactured by site sponsors.[54] In contrast, most public sector sites accept no commercial advertising or offer products on a for-profit basis.[55] Consumer concerns about the accuracy and quality of health care information, especially on commercial sites, limit public use of and confidence in these resources.

Some studies have questioned the reliability and accuracy of medical information stored on electronic devices. A research project by Eysenbach and colleagues, for example, shows that medical websites vary enormously in the validity of their online information.[56] Although the amount of accessible information has risen dramatically in recent years, there are few content standards. Some information is incomplete or inaccurate, or it is sponsored by pharmaceutical interests with a financial stake in particular treatments.

Potential conflicts of interest are important because national surveys have found that 75 percent of Americans report that they rarely check the source or date of medical resources found online.[57] Internet users are apt to take what they see online at face value instead of doing any fact checking or raising questions about the objectivity of the material viewed. Such behavior restricts consumers' ability to derive full benefits from digital information sources.

In addition, disturbing variations exist in website quality by sponsorship status. Private sector sites have the highest level of real or potential conflicts of interest because they are sponsored by for-profit entities, such as medical equipment and pharmaceutical manufacturers. We

demonstrate that it is difficult for private site visitors to protect themselves from self-interested medical advice or commercial advertising
because of the way in which the information is presented on these sites.
For example, it often is difficult to distinguish impartial advice from
sponsored links.

Private sites also are more likely than public sector sites to follow
niche strategies. Rather than seeking to serve all constituents, for-profit
sites focus on particular illnesses that offer them the opportunity to make
money or on expensive prescription drugs manufactured by site sponsors. That means that medical information found online must be taken
with great caution.

Privacy Concerns

A final problem that constrains technology adoption is worry about
privacy and security issues related to the use of electronic devices.
According to survey data, many Americans are concerned about the confidentiality of online medical information,[58] and 62 percent of adults in
a recent national poll felt that use of electronic medical records makes it
more difficult to ensure patients' privacy.[59] Seventy-five percent of Internet users worried that health care websites would share their personal
information without their permission.[60]

A significant percentage of web visitors said that they do not take
advantage of online medical resources because of fear that their information will be compromised. Forty percent said they will not give a doctor online access to their medical records, 25 percent said that they will
not buy online prescriptions, and 16 percent said that they will not register at medical websites. Overall, 17 percent refused to seek medical
advice online due to privacy fears. Nearly 80 percent claimed that a
detailed privacy policy would improve their interest in taking advantage
of online medical resources.[61]

Americans fear that confidential information stored on digital devices
will be compromised and communicated to others. While those fears also
exist with regard to paper records, the concern about electronic information makes people less willing to adopt digital records and use them
to store sensitive information. A Pew Internet and American Life Project
found that 85 percent of U.S. consumers fear that their health insurance
company might raise their rates if the company discovers what health
care websites they have visited. Sixty-three percent believe that placing
medical records online is "a bad thing," even if the material is protected

by a security password.[62] Seventeen percent of people in a Harris Interactive survey reported that they withhold information from medical personnel due to concerns that those individuals would disclose the data to others without unauthorizztion.[63]

Research has found that security breaches of computerized information are more common in the United States than in Europe.[64] Many European nations have strict privacy laws that protect patient confidentiality, but the United States has a patchwork of state and federal rules that are not always effective in doing so. Data collection is a growth industry in the United States, with a number of firms such as ChoicePoint and Acxiom selling people's private information. Commercial firms in Europe face many more restrictions on their ability to compile information without someone's personal consent.[65]

OUTLINE OF THE STUDY

In order to evaluate the claims of health information advocates, it is important to collect empirical data regarding online content, sponsorship status, public usage, the relationship between use of e-health information sources and attitudes about health care, and experiences with technology outside the United States. Digital medicine is an area in which claims often are made without adequate testing of key propositions. Only by having basic knowledge about the supply and demand sides of digital medicine is it possible to understand the realistic potential for electronic health.

This research relies on several original data sources to investigate the promise and benefits of health information technology. One source is a November 2005 national telephone survey of 928 Americans eighteen years of age or older (see appendix A for poll methodology and questions) that assesses use of health care technology, disparities among different social and economic groups, and obstacles to use of information technology in the health care arena.

Using results from this survey, we compare use of conventional in-person and telephone interactions with physicians and other health care providers with use of digital communication strategies such as e-mail contact with providers, health website visits, and online purchases of prescription drugs and other medical products. We find that most people feel more comfortable using conventional personal and phone-based interactions than health information technology, and we document disparities in health-related Internet use by region and by user's socio-economic status and attitude. We also assess potential reasons and strategies for addressing prevailing disparities.

We employ a national survey because the public perspective is important to the future of digital medicine. How people feel about technology, what drives their reactions, and what obstacles they see to the use of health information technology are crucial. Aggregate studies of technology use that compare it with health outcomes cannot assess an individual's experiences and motivations. Even when clear positive or negative relationships exist, it is not clear why they develop. One of the virtues of public surveys is that they let researchers discern why people feel the way that they do and determine what would induce them to make greater use of information technology than they currently do. That is especially important given the worries that many Americans have expressed about online security and privacy.

Whether people who rely on digital resources have attitudes and behaviors that differ from those of people who do not is an important question. Rather than accept the word of technology advocates, it is crucial to investigate the impact of digital medicine on consumers. Is there any association between type of interaction with health care professionals and how people judge quality, access, or affordability? For example, are those who visit websites, communicate electronically with doctors, or order medications online any more likely to say that they experience good quality health care that is affordable and accessible? Surveys allow us to investigate those perceptions and link them to demographic background and social and political variables.

If there is no difference in attitudes between those using digital and conventional medical care, it casts doubt on whether electronic health technology can deliver the benefits claimed by its advocates. E-health must offer the hope of improved services and cheaper medical care; it makes little sense to invest substantial resources in technology innovation otherwise. It costs large amounts of money to create electronic medical records, build the broadband infrastructure necessary for maintaining quality websites, and devise two-way communications systems between doctors and patients. Digital medicine needs to provide benefits greater than those provided by the current system in order to justify the upfront costs of implementing new technology. Policymakers need to know what the greatest benefits are as they consider alternative strategies for promoting technological innovation.

To assess the impact of site sponsorship, we analyze the content of government, commercial, and nonprofit health websites. We focus in particular on the kind of information and services online, potential or real conflicts of interest in the material provided, and the extent to which sites can be accessed by disabled people, those who are not proficient in the English language, and those with low literacy. This part of our study investigates health department websites maintained by the fifty U.S. state governments as well as the most popular commercial and nonprofit sites (see appendix B for the list of U.S. websites examined). In particular, we are interested in how health websites maintained by nongovernment entities handle advertising, sponsorship disclosure, access for people with disabilities and those who do not understand the language, and readability (see appendix D for details on the content analysis).

We use Watchfire WebXM software to evaluate the accessibility of websites for those who have physical impairments (especially those who are visually impaired) and the Flesch-Kincaid readability test employed by the U.S. Department of Defense to determine whether websites are written at a grade level that those with limited literacy can understand. We check to see what languages are represented on health websites as a means of evaluating non-native speakers' access to information. We search sites to determine the quality of privacy or security policies and whether they prohibit commercial marketing of visitor information; use of cookies, which automatically create electronic profiles of website visitors; disclosure of personal information without prior consent of the visitor; and disclosure of visitor information to law enforcement agents. We suggest remedies based on our findings that will improve the accessibility, privacy, and security of health information posted online.

Finally, to study global political and social dynamics, we present a content analysis of national government health departments around the world (see appendix C) and non-U.S. case studies of health information technology to determine what works and what does not in the area of health information technology. The content analysis looks at the same considerations as in the U.S. study. We study websites to see how they handle privacy and security, whether sites can be accessed by people with physical impairments and non-native speakers, and whether sites accept commercial advertising.

Using non-U.S. examples, we study how officials in various countries have implemented health information technology. Asian and European countries, for example, have placed a tremendous amount of health information online using high-speed broadband technology that allows them to read X-rays, CT scans, and other materials included in electronic health records at a distance, thereby improving the speed and quality of health care delivery. We draw on those experiences to help understand innovations in delivery of health care information in a variety of political, social, and economic settings and to compare the U.S. experience with that in other countries.

By looking at survey data, website content information, and case studies of successful use of technology, we seek to understand where the United States is in the technology revolution and what steps need to be taken in order to extend the benefits of digital medicine to all people. Right now, numerous obstacles need to be overcome. Through better understanding of the e-health revolution, it will be possible to move rapidly into the future and overcome many of the barriers that currently exist.

CHAPTER TWO

Online Content and Sponsorship Status

Visitors to the Pennsylvania Department of Health can scan holdings in a medical information clearinghouse that covers major diseases, access a list of available visiting nurses, and submit forms to register for courses on emergency medical services. The Massachusetts Department of Health and Human Services allows people to use electronic forms to determine their eligibility for assistance programs, request American Sign Language interpreters, renew professional licenses, file medical claims, and see data on health care providers. States such as California, New York, and Michigan post data online so that residents can compare the quality and performance of hospitals, physicians, and nursing homes.[1]

On most of these public sector sites there are no commercial ads, sponsored links, or product placements. It is clear that a government agency sponsors the site. Visitors understand when they visit these sites that the information providers are not seeking to make money and do not want to sell them anything; their purpose is to provide up-to-date material on whatever is relevant to the public mission of their agency.

The contrast with commercial and nonprofit health sites could not be starker. Visitors to WebMD.com, About.com, and other private sites see material regarding specific illnesses and have the option to order medication from online drug pharmacies. But in looking for information on diseases and illnesses, patients are bombarded with ads, video clips, sponsored links, and targeted appeals. Sponsorship is less clear on commercial sites, and some push products linked to the corporate interests that finance the sites.

It has been estimated that there are more than 100,000 websites devoted to health-related subjects;[2] they range from official government websites to those of nonprofit organizations and commercial sites sponsored by pharmaceutical companies. WebMD.com and About.com have become popular places to go for medical information. Google Health, Microsoft, and RevolutionHealth.com (started by former America Online founder Stephen Case) meanwhile have developed new portals that offer consumers information on health and fitness. These sites allow anyone with or even without medical knowledge to become a "contributor" and write pages that they deem helpful for medical care.[3]

In comparing commercial websites with those in the public sector, it becomes apparent that they have different incentives for online content, advertising, and access.[4] Private sites are more likely than public ones to engage in niche strategies focusing on prominent illnesses and to have site sponsors selling products that they manufacture. They furthermore rely much more substantially than government sites on commercial advertising and are less likely to be accessible to non–English speakers and those with physical impairments. That makes commercial sites less available to underserved groups and exposes patients to real or potential conflicts of interest.[5]

There also can be withholding of damaging information or conflicts of interest in the presentation of medical data at for-profit websites. During a lawsuit over one of its antidepressant drugs, Avandia, the drug company GlaxoSmithKline posted clinical trial data online for various pharmaceuticals. Independent researchers reanalyzed the data and in an article published in the *New England Journal of Medicine* claimed that "Avandia posed a heightened cardiac risk." Their discovery led to calls for legislation requiring drug manufacturers to disclose clinical trial results.[6]

This chapter evaluates the online content of government, commercial, and nonprofit health care websites. We use a detailed content analysis of health department websites maintained by the fifty state governments from 2000 to 2007; a 2007 study of the content of the forty-four most popular commercial websites, as judged by the Nielsen/Net Ratings; and a 2007 analysis of the thirty top nonprofit sites, as determined by the Medical Library Association. (See appendix B for the list of sites involved in each analysis.) We investigate interactive features, online reports and databases, readability level, accessibility for non–English speakers, accessibility for disabled users, commercial advertising, sponsorship disclosure, and the presence of privacy and security statements.

In general, we show that private websites offer a wealth of medical information but are more likely than public sites to have ads, create real or perceived conflicts of interest, and have weak disclosure of site sponsors, limiting their overall utility to health care consumers. Since national public opinion surveys demonstrate that people are twice as likely to visit a private as a public site, the contrasts between public and private sites show the risks facing those who rely primarily on commercial locations.

WEBSITE QUALITY

Having strong website quality standards is crucial to the future of public use of electronic health resources. According to federal authorities, two-thirds of Americans who use the Internet for health care information have problems evaluating the accuracy of electronic sources.[7] Only 20 percent of patients say that they are able to find all the information that they need when they search the web.[8] The wide variety of site sponsors, the different ways in which information is presented, and variations in use of ads and sponsored links is confusing to ordinary users. Such lack of clarity regarding site sponsors or sources of information presented complicates individuals' ability to rate the reliability of the online information that they review.[9]

Such aspects of digital sources of medical information make it difficult to know which sites contain objective, authoritative advice. There is tremendous variation in the content and design of online medical sites. Some feature interactive services, while others function more as static billboards of health information. It is not always clear what a site's orientation is. Some sites do not present themselves as commercial in nature even when they are, and most seek to raise their visibility and traffic level by appearing to present clear, objective, and noncommercial information. Some for-profit sites even masquerade as nonprofit sites through unclear disclosure of their sponsors.

To help consumers judge online information, policy advocates have proposed adoption of a code of conduct for web portals. The Health on the Net Foundation (HON) is one organization that has developed guidelines for presenting information that cover authoritativeness (information should be given by medical professionals), complementarity (information should supplement, not replace, the physician-patient relationship), confidentiality (site security and privacy should be maintained), attribution (sources should have appropriate references), justifiability (proper evidence should be presented), transparency of authorship and sponsorship (authors and sponsors should be clearly identified), and honesty in advertising and editorial policy (ads and original content should be clearly differentiated).[10]

Websites that meet those standards are allowed to place the HON seal of approval—designed to be similar to the Good Housekeeping Seal of Approval—on the site. That tells consumers that certain sites meet high standards of website quality and that they can trust the information that those sites present. So far, however, few commercial health-related sites have acquired the HON seal of approval, indicating that most are unable to guarantee that their information is clear, authoritative, transparent, and honest.

Other observers have pointed out the importance of accessibility and readability on health websites. One study of English- and Spanish-language medical websites found that the reading level required to comprehend the material completely is too high for the average person. For example, all of the English-language sites and 86 percent of the Spanish-language sites examined required the user to have at least high school reading ability, which far exceeds the reading proficiency of many Americans.

In addition, much of the information found on the sites included inaccuracies or was incomplete.[11] Some sites had material that was out of date, misleading, or downright dangerous to health care consumers.[12] In the world of digital medicine, it is crucial for consumers of online information to be aware of what they are reading and to evaluate material very carefully in order to protect their own well-being.

DISCLOSURE OF SPONSORS

Nearly all health care websites disclose the sponsor of the page. With state government sites, it is obvious that the site is operated by the public sector; these sites feature the state emblem and offer links to official government agencies. Meanwhile, nonpublic—commercial or nonprofit—sites feature an "About Us" link that tells the user what entity sponsors the site and what its activities are.

However, with nonpublic sites, the level of detail in the disclosure is weak. We identified three levels of detail: a little, some, or a lot of detail. "A little" means that the site listed the name, address, and phone number of the sponsor; "some" means that the site provided information regarding the sponsor's activities; and "a lot" means that the site included material on what the sponsor has done, what its goals are, who its contributors are, and what its products are.

None of the commercial or nonprofit sites investigated were categorized as providing "a lot" of detail. Sixty-eight percent of commercial sites and 17 percent of nonprofits fell within the category of "a little" detail, while 32 percent of commercial sites and 83 percent of nonprofit sites offered "some" disclosure. Most disclosure statements offered minimal information, such as name and address, but not much material on organizational goals, activities, or purposes.

For example, the About Us section for WebMD.com is buried near the bottom of a page containing a large number of medical links. Its statement offers little information about who operates the site and forces visitors to go to other places for information on contributors. As quoted here in full, the disclosure statement leaves much to be desired:

> The WebMD content staff blends award-winning expertise in medicine, journalism, health communication and content creation to bring you the best health information possible. Our esteemed colleagues at MedicineNet.com are frequent contributors to WebMD and comprise our Medical Editorial Board. Our Independent Medical Review Board continuously reviews the site for accuracy and timeliness.

Despite the appearance of openness in this statement, the link to MedicineNet.com is not clickable, which means visitors must exit WebMD.com and independently enter the URL of that site to view it. That additional step may be enough to discourage many people from linking to the disclosure material. When visitors cannot click through to a new website, they generally get frustrated and do not pursue additional information. On accessing MedicineNet.com's About Us section, which is located on a crowded page, visitors find the following information:

> MedicineNet.com is an online, healthcare media publishing company. It provides easy-to-read, in-depth, authoritative medical

information for consumers via its robust, user-friendly, interactive web site. Since 1996, MedicineNet.com has had a highly accomplished, uniquely experienced team of qualified executives in the fields of medicine, healthcare, Internet technology, and business to bring you the most comprehensive, sought-after healthcare information anywhere. Nationally recognized, doctor-produced by a network of over 70 U.S. board certified physicians, Medicine Net.com is the trusted source for online health and medical information. The doctors of MedicineNet are also proud to author *Webster's New World(tm) Medical Dictionary*, first and second editions (January 2003), John Wiley & Sons, Inc.; ISBN: 0-7645-2461-5. MedicineNet, Inc.'s main office is in San Clemente, California, and the corporate office is in New York, New York. Please reference www.wbmd.com for corporate information.

Only by clicking on wbmd.com does one find information on the company's board of directors and management team, but little information is given on what the corporation does.

The information included in the About Us links notes that WebMD. com and MedicineNet.com are corporate entities that publish information online that is developed by executives in the fields of medicine, health care, Internet technology, and business. But they provide no details on who those individuals are or what their financial interests are. The site offers virtually no guidance to consumers interested in details about site sponsors, only statements of generic content that are not helpful in evaluating the accuracy, objectivity, or fairness of the material presented.

Weak disclosure of sponsors on WebMD.com and other commercial sites makes it difficult for consumers to determine who is behind them. Visitors do not receive basic information regarding the commercial interests of site sponsors and how those interests might affect the medical advice presented or products pushed on the site. Having little or no background information is risky for consumers because they have no way to evaluate the real or potential conflicts of interest that may exist on such websites.

ACCESSIBILITY

Accessibility is a major goal of U.S. policymakers. Legally, equity in access to government services is mandated for particular groups, such as physically impaired individuals (through the U.S. Rehabilitation Act) and racial minorities (through equal opportunity legislation). There also is social and political pressure for policymakers to provide equitable access; for example, advocacy groups representing people with low education or low literacy as well as non–English speakers lobby to ensure fair access to medical information.[13] Finally, there are economic incentives for improving access. In order to reach the economies of scale necessary to make technology cost effective, governments need to boost the number of website visitors. Anything that limits traffic weakens the long-term economic rationale for electronic government.

One key aspect of accessibility involves disability. U.S. census figures indicate that 49.7 million Americans have a long-lasting physical impairment. That figure includes 9.3 million with a disability that involves sight or hearing; 21.2 million with a condition that limits basic physical activities; 12.4 million with a physical, mental, or emotional condition that limits their ability to learn or remember; 6.8 million with a condition that interferes with their ability to dress or bathe themselves; and 18.2 million with a condition that makes it difficult for them to leave their homes.[14]

Given the fact that 19.3 percent of the U.S. population suffers from one or more physical impairments, it is critical that government web designers ensure the accessibility of e-health resources regardless of user disabilities related to sight, hearing, or movement. In order to determine how accessible state health websites are for the physically impaired, we employed Watchfire's automated software on usability (known as "Bobby"), which scans websites for a number of features designed to improve usability for people with different kinds of impairments.

For example, it is crucial to have appropriate color contrasts in website texts and backgrounds so that visually impaired people can read what is on the computer screen. In addition, it is important to have text-equivalent "alt" tags on images so that software used by the visually impaired that converts text to audio signals recognizes that a picture of the U.S. Capitol (or any other object) is of that building (or object).

For individuals with hearing impairments, websites need to display procedures for using Text Telephones (TYY) or Telecommunications Devices for the Deaf (TDD), tools that allow deaf individuals to communicate with government officials through text display devices. They require agencies to have designated telephone lines so that when hearing impaired people call, both parties have access to TYY/TDD machines.

For those with limited mobility, data tables need to be written in a clear and hierarchical way so that software programs can make sense of online information. Specialized software for individuals with mobility impairments helps them navigate complex databases and documents, for example, through voice commands or eye movements. Failure to have well-designed website features may drive potential users away and limit user traffic at a health site.

We took the attributes identified by Watchfire's "Bobby" software and applied the priority level one standard recommended by the World Wide Web Consortium (W3C) in assessing the websites. The minimum standard for website accessibility recommended by disability advocates, it checks for compliance with a variety of accessibility features such as text equivalents for audio, video, or pictures; the ability to output text to Braille displays or speech synthesizers; use of appropriate color backgrounds, markup, and style sheets that convey the layout and structure of text and data; and adaptability to voice commands or to head and eye movements. We judged both public and private health websites to be either in compliance or not in compliance.

Our findings reveal improvement in accessibility over time. In 2003, 30 percent of the state health department sites met the W3C accessibility test, and the percentage increased over time, to 40 percent in 2004; 42 percent in 2005 and 2006; and 52 percent in 2007. However, the results show that more than twice as many public sites as private sites were deemed to be accessible. In 2007, only 18 percent of commercial sites and 13 percent of nonprofit sites were accessible, while 52 percent of public sector sites were.

The higher degree of accessibility for disabled individuals on public sites demonstrates greater justice and equity in access to public e-health resources. Commercial sites are set up to make money, and they do not have the same incentives as government agencies to help underserved populations. That clearly limits the benefits of electronic health resources for millions of individuals with visual, hearing, or physical impairments; as a result, many of the people who have the greatest need for up-to-date medical information are least able to share the advantages of online sources.

Language accessibility represents another crucial dimension of website accessibility. When 17.9 percent of the U.S. population speaks a language other than English at home, the ability of these individuals to make use of e-health resources becomes an issue. In some parts of the country, the portion of the population that does not speak English rises to more than one-third. For example, 39.5 percent of residents in California and 36.5 percent of those who live in New Mexico speak a non-English language at home.[15]

The presence of so many people in the United States who do not speak English represents a major challenge for health care providers. It is difficult for medical professionals to communicate with them and for them to comprehend health care information, whether presented in person or over the Internet. For something as important and personal as health care, clear communication is vital. Patients need to understand nuances of meaning related to medical treatment and diagnosis.

To evaluate language accessibility, we looked at whether health websites provided information in languages other than English. In 2000, only 10 percent of state health sites provided any kind of non-English materials. The numbers were not much better over the next two years. In 2001, 8 percent of state health department sites offered translations of English-language materials; 10 percent did so in 2002.

However, the number of sites providing translations rose thereafter. In 2003, 32 percent of state health websites had medical information in languages other than English. That number increased to 44 percent in 2004 but dropped down to 34 percent in 2005 as some agencies took some foreign language materials offline for security reasons, such as material about anthrax or other dangerous organisms or contaminants. In 2006, 76 percent of sites provided translations; in 2007, 44 percent did so.

Commercial sites fared much worse on the dimension of language accessibility. Only 16 percent of for-profit health websites provided translations, well below the level of government websites. The low level of language accessibility on commercial sites demonstrates the relative lack of interest these health information providers have in serving non-English-speaking populations. Since some of these people are poor or are not in a position to take advantage of electronic resources because of lack of access to computers and digital technology, businesses do not pay much attention to them.

In contrast, nonprofit sites do much better than commercial sites on language accessibility. Fifty-seven percent of nonprofit sites offer translations, similar to the percentage of public sector health sites. Because they have a broader mission than commercial sites, they take more seriously the task of helping those in need of language assistance to understand the information that they present.

The poor numbers for commercial websites suggest that businesses have a long way to go before equal access is available. At the national level, statutes dealing with federal elections require that communities with any non-English-speaking population exceeding 5 percent must provide ballots in the native language of that group.[16] In the same spirit, government agencies mandate equal access for those with physical impairments. If the principle of equal access were applied to health information, many websites would flunk the accessibility standard established by the federal government in other areas.

READABILITY

Literacy is the ability to read and understand written information. According to national statistics, about half of the U.S. population reads at the eighth-grade level or lower.[17] Not only is that a general problem, but there also are troubling differences in literacy by race, gender, education, and income. Minorities, women, and those of limited education and income typically have more difficulty comprehending the written word than their counterparts.[18]

Poor literacy is a particular concern in the area of health due to the sensitivity of medical information and the importance of good health to quality of life and general well-being. As health sites place more information and services online, electronic resources need to be understandable by a wide range of consumers. That imperative is especially salient given growing evidence documenting significant health illiteracy and its relationship to cost and quality of medical care and access to it.[19] Healthy People 2010 defines health literacy as "the degree to which individuals have the capacity to obtain, process, and understand basic health information and services needed to make appropriate health decisions."[20] If information on official health websites is written at too high a level for visitors to comprehend, online technology will not reach its full potential as a public health information tool.

Failure to write documents in an understandable manner makes it more difficult for officials to address social, political, and economic inequities. A number of researchers have evaluated various forms of written communications—such as warning labels, brochures, forms, and instructions—to see whether they are written at a reasonable level. Results indicate that pamphlets and educational materials frequently are too complicated for the populations that they target to understand.

TABLE 2-1. Health-Related Websites by Readability Level
Percent of sites

Readability level	Government sites					Commercial sites	Nonprofit sites
	2003	2004	2005	2006	2007	2007	2007
Fourth grade or less	2	12	10	2	6	2	10
Fifth grade	2	2	2	2	0	7	0
Sixth grade	2	0	0	2	0	7	3
Seventh grade	0	2	4	7	4	11	7
Eighth grade	0	0	4	4	6	23	7
Ninth grade	4	10	6	7	8	11	10
Tenth grade	8	12	8	4	10	11	10
Eleventh grade	12	12	4	0	12	7	7
Twelfth grade or more	70	50	62	72	54	21	46
Mean grade level	11.2	10.6	10.9	10.7	11.4	8.7	9.6

Source: Authors' e-health content analysis, 2003–07.

Indeed, a review of 216 published articles on health literacy by the Council on Scientific Affairs found widespread evidence of health illiteracy and clear links between poor literacy and inadequate understanding of medical treatments.[21] Often, research has found racial disparities and other types of class-based barriers to comprehension of medical information.[22] Although Medicaid enrollees read at approximately the fifth-grade level, most health care information is written at the tenth-grade level or higher.[23]

To see whether such findings hold up for public e-health resources, we examined public and nonpublic health websites to test the readability, by grade level, of the front page of each site. We employed the Flesch-Kincaid test, a standard tool for evaluating readability that is used by the U.S. Department of Defense. It computes readability by dividing average sentence length (number of words divided by number of sentences) by the average number of syllables per word (number of syllables divided by the number of words).[24] Its central premise is that if all citizens are to fully understand what they read, sentence structure and word usage cannot be too complicated.

As shown in table 2-1, the average readability of state health websites was at the grade 11.2 level in 2003, grade 10.6 level in 2004, grade 10.9 level in 2005, grade 10.7 level in 2006, and grade 11.4 level in 2007. The readability of 70 percent of sites in 2003, 50 percent in 2004, 62 percent

TABLE 2-2. Health-Related Websites Providing Publications, Data, and Services
Percent of sites

Option provided	Government sites								Com-mercial sites 2007	Non-profit sites 2007
	2000	2001	2002	2003	2004	2005	2006	2007		
Publications	88	98	98	100	100	98	100	100	91	97
Data	42	72	64	98	98	94	94	100	91	100
Audio clips	6	2	0	6	16	4	28	26	30	40
Video clips	4	4	6	2	18	16	38	46	50	40
Online services	20	36	20	48	68	92	92	98	96	100
Credit card payment	4	24	10	28	36	76	66	74	43	40

Source: Authors' e-health content analysis, 2000–07.

in 2005, 72 percent in 2006, and 54 percent in 2007 was at the twelfth-grade level. The readability of only 6 percent of sites in 2003, 16 percent in 2004, 20 percent in 2005, 17 percent in 2006, and 16 percent in 2007 fell at the eighth-grade level or below, which is the reading level of half of the U.S. public.

Those numbers are worse than those for nonpublic sites. The readability of commercial health websites was at an average grade level of 8.7 in 2007, and the mean level for nonprofit sites was 9.6. Only 21 percent of commercial sites and 46 percent of nonprofit sites were written at the twelfth-grade level. Most fell significantly closer to the reading level of ordinary Americans.

Based on this analysis, it is obvious that many health sites are written well above the reading level of the typical American, especially on government and nonprofit sites. Commercial sites do relatively better because they want to sell products and have a clear incentive to make sure visitors understand the material that they present. They want people to acquire timely health information and have access to online medical services.

CONTENT AND SERVICES

We also analyzed the content of health websites. From our analysis, it is evident that both public and private sites have placed a wide variety of publications, data, and services online. As shown in table 2-2, nearly all websites offer publications and databases, and most provide online services. In the public sector, common services include the option to compare the performance of hospitals, find medical professionals, and order reports.

On commercial and nonprofit sites, visitors can order medications, ask questions, and seek professional care. For example, sites such as WebMD.com allow users to spot the warning signs of skin cancer and learn how to assess their "sleep personality." After watching videos or slideshows, people can access ads that provide pharmaceutical or alternative remedies to particular maladies. Private sites are more likely to be media rich and to offer audio and video clips. Because consumers like to receive information in a nontext, visual form, having health materials in video format is a good marketing strategy. However, public sector health departments are more likely to feature the ability to pay for online purchases by credit card. States are placing more and more services online, and that makes it easy for patients to pay for the desired services.

INTERACTIVITY

Commercial and nonprofit sites are more likely than government websites to offer interactive features. For example, technology is available that allows websites to provide updates electronically through newsletters, e-mail messages, and magazines to people who register their interests in particular areas. It also is possible to tailor website information to the personal interests of visitors and to access websites not just through desktop or laptop computers but through mobile devices such as cell phones or personal digital assistants (PDAs).

Except for e-mail, public sector sites have been less likely than nonpublic ones to embrace interactive technologies (see table 2-3). Eighty-two percent of commercial sites and 67 percent of nonprofit sites offer electronic updates, while only 38 percent of state health departments do so. In 2007, website personalization was available from 82 percent of commercial sites and 50 percent of nonprofit sites but only 4 percent of public sites. Fourteen percent of commercial sites, 23 percent of nonprofit sites, and 0 percent of public sites provide PDA access.

PRIVACY AND SECURITY

Privacy and security are major concerns of many web users. In a national survey undertaken by the nonprofit Council for Excellence in Government,

TABLE 2-3. Health-Related Sites Offering Interactive Features
Percent of sites

Feature	Government sites								Com-mercial sites	Non-profit sites
	2000	2001	2002	2003	2004	2005	2006	2007	2007	2007
E-mail	64	84	88	92	94	86	98	96	91	80
Comments	24	0	8	24	32	26	56	48	64	67
Updates	4	4	6	8	14	14	38	38	82	67
Personalization	2	2	2	0	2	6	0	4	82	50
PDA access	--	--	--	0	0	0	0	0	14	23

Source: Authors' e-health content analysis, 2000–07.

confidentiality was at the top of the list of problems that Americans had with government websites.[25] People expressed fear over the privacy of online transactions and threats to confidential information stored online. The most negative worries that citizens had about e-government were about terrorists making use of online information (32 percent), users having less personal privacy (24 percent), hackers breaking into personal computers (19 percent), and people without Internet service getting less government service (13 percent).[26] Those fears need to be taken seriously. If citizens do not have confidence in public websites, they are not likely to make use of the electronic resources that they offer.[27]

Privacy issues are of special concern in the area of health because of the sensitivity of medical data. With the increasing number of online transactions on government health websites, citizens fear security breaches that will compromise their confidential information. Well-publicized unauthorized disclosures at some medical establishments have intensified concerns, placing privacy and security center stage in the e-health debate among the general public.[28]

A study of popular health sites revealed that the privacy policies of many fall short of the public's desired standards. Most statements did not meet minimum standards, such as by "providing adequate notice, giving users some control over their information, and holding the sites' business partners to the same privacy standards."[29] National surveys find that visitors say that they are less willing to provide personal information on websites that have marketing partners (88 percent), that automatically collect information through cookies (79 percent), that are sponsored by an insurance company (45 percent) or a pharmaceutical

TABLE 2-4. Health-Related Sites Having Privacy and Security Policies
Percent of sites

| Policy | Government sites | | | | | | | | Com-mercial sites | Non-profit sites |
	2000	2001	2002	2003	2004	2005	2006	2007	2007	2007
Privacy	8	32	46	68	76	86	78	88	98	77
Security	4	22	38	46	50	62	68	56	84	40

Source: Authors' e-health content analysis, 2000–07.

company (40 percent), or that are promoted in national television adver-tisements (19 percent).[30] Since many commercial sites feature one or more of those characteristics, public concerns about the privacy and security of electronic information online are understandable.

As shown in table 2-4, there have been major improvements in the provision on state health department websites of privacy and security statements outlining how those concerns are addressed. In 2000, only 8 percent of health departments had an online privacy policy and only 4 percent had a security policy. However, by 2007, the numbers had grown to 88 percent for privacy policies and 56 percent for security policies. Nearly all commercial sites and 77 percent of nonprofit sites offer pri-vacy policies, and 84 percent of commercial sites and 40 percent of non-profit websites provide security policies.

We also examined health department privacy policies. Among the issues considered important in this area are whether the privacy state-ment prohibits commercial marketing of visitor information, use of indi-vidual profiles or "cookies" to identify visitors, disclosure of personal information without the prior consent of the visitor, or disclosure of vis-itor information to law enforcement agents. Prohibition of such practices keeps consumers from being bombarded with "spam" and from having their online movements monitored through digital technology.

Our analysis found major improvements over the last few years (see table 2-5). In 2001, only 14 percent of state health websites prohibited the commercial marketing of information provided by visitors, 16 per-cent prohibited cookies, and 12 percent banned the sharing of personal information without prior consent. However, by 2005, 82 percent had policies prohibiting the commercial marketing of visitor information, 26 percent prohibited the use of cookies or individual profiles, and 80 per-cent said that they did not share personal information, a marked increase

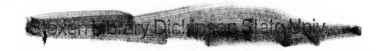

TABLE 2-5. Provisions of Health-Related Website Privacy Statements
Percent of sites

Policy	Government sites							Commercial sites	Non-profit sites
	2001	2002	2003	2004	2005	2006	2007	2007	2007
Prohibits commercial marketing	14	48	42	52	82	68	76	77	70
Prohibits cookies	16	4	16	18	26	20	42	0	20
Prohibits sharing of personal information	12	42	44	38	80	64	44	77	60
Permits sharing of personal information with law enforcement agencies	. . .	40	44	42	76	50	54	96	57

Source: Authors' e-health content analysis, 2000–07.

from 38 percent during the previous year. That is in contrast with the 76 percent of sites that said that they could disclose visitor information to law enforcement agents, up from 42 percent a year earlier. The substantial increase in states willing to disclose information to law enforcement agencies reflects, in part, additional security measures implemented in the wake of the Patriot Act and the report of the 9-11 Commission.

Nonpublic sites do well on several privacy dimensions. Seventy-seven percent of commercial sites and 70 percent of nonprofit sites prohibit the commercial marketing of visitor information, while 77 percent of commercial sites and 60 percent of nonprofit sites prohibit sharing of personal information obtained during site visits. However, commercial sites do poorly on use of cookies. None of the for-profit sites and only 20 percent of the nonprofit sites prohibit use of cookies, which allows websites to compile and store information on visitors and employ that material for their own purposes.

COMMERCIAL ADVERTISING

Few state health department websites feature commercial advertising. Overall, less than 4 percent of sites studied between 2000 and 2007 had product ads, and many did not have user fees to access particular services or information. There were few ads because government jurisdictions did not want conflicts of interest to arise with respect to the health

TABLE 2-6. Health-Related Websites Having Commercial Advertising and User Fees
Percent of sites

Policy	Government sites								Commercial sites 2007	Nonprofit sites 2007
	2000	2001	2002	2003	2004	2005	2006	2007		
Ads	4	0	0	0	18	0	0	2	61	17
Fees	...	...	2	4	42	4	52	48	9	10

Source: Authors' e-health content analysis, 2000–07.

information that they place online (see table 2-6). Policymakers understand that the public arena is not a place where private companies should be hawking their products or services. Since most government agencies do not feature product endorsements, it is not surprising that we find few ads on public sector sites. Just as people would be shocked to find an ad for a headache or upset stomach remedy in a health department building, they do not want to see pharmaceutical commercials at government websites.

However, 61 percent of commercial sites and 17 percent of nonprofit sites have product ads, and some charge user fees. Advertisements range from plugs for pharmaceuticals to spots on treatment at weight-loss clinics and hospitals. Fifty-two of the commercial sites and 53 percent of nonprofit sites feature ads from the sponsor of the site. That means that these sites are embedding advertisements from their own sponsors within the medical advice that they offer.

In addition, many sites engage in targeting needy patients. For example, 27 percent of commercial sites are designed for specific groups, such as the poor, elderly, or disabled or those having particular diseases. Even nonprofit sites are not immune; 30 percent of them target particular groups. That means that those who are most vulnerable to commercial marketing are the ones most exposed to advertising appeals.

To demonstrate the prevalence of advertising on commercial sites, we studied ads on three of the most popular health sites: WebMD.com, About.com, and MayoClinic.org. In June 2007, when we examined the sites, WebMD had sixteen text ads, twenty banner ads, and twelve links to medical ads supplied by Google.com. Figure 2-1 lists a selection of the ads. One can see that most were in the medical and health area, but there

FIGURE 2-1. WebMD Ads

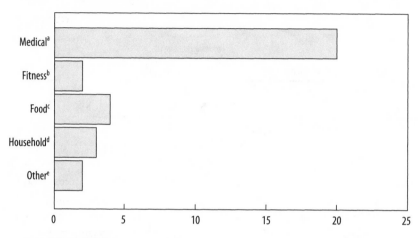

Source: Authors' compilation.

a. *Prontix* (acid reflux disease); *Seroquel* (bipolar disorder) by AstraZeneca; *Actonel* (bone health); *Mederma for Kids;* *Herceptin* (breast cancer) by Genentech; *Enbrel* (clearer skin) by Amgen; *Enablex* (overactive bladder) by Novartis; *Rituxan* (RA support) by Genentech; *Aricept* (Alzheimer's) by Eisai and Exelon; pain relief medication by the Stryker Corporation; various cancer treatments by AstraZeneca; knee pain treatments by Zimmer; asthma medication by Genentech and by Novartis; skin care treatments by Unilever; MS LifeLines; cardiac device videos from Saint Jude Medical Center; *Tylenol* by McNeil; *St. Joseph's Aspirin* by McNeil; *Claritin* by Schering-Plough.

b. WebMD Weight Loss Clinic; Nebraska Medical Center.

c. *Minute Maid* enhanced juices; *Applebees;* *Splenda* brand sweetener; *Smart Start* cereal by Kellogg's.

d. *Colgate* toothpaste; *Secret* antiperspirant by Proctor and Gamble; *Huggies* diapers.

e. *Quest* minivan by Nissan's; The Biggest Loser Club.

also were ads for fitness, food, household, and other products. In addition, there were a variety of sponsored Google Ad links such as www.MassGeneral.org/Cancer, www.easyweightlosstea.com, www.skincareRX.com, www.bestpricetanning.com, and www.thefootdoctor.com.

About.com featured fifty-two display ads, which spanned the gauntlet of medical, fitness, food, household, and other products (see figure 2-2). The site also included sponsored Google Ad links such as www.TheOrthopedicSite.com, www.kneereplacement.com, www.BrighamAndWomens.org, and www.RevolutionHealth.com. The site included "Offers," a feature that provides hundreds of sponsored links to specific diseases and conditions. According to the website, "These offers are linked to ads purchased by companies that want to advertise next to relevant content, based on a set of keywords they specify. The offers are administered, sorted, and maintained by a third party."

FIGURE 2-2. About.Com Ads

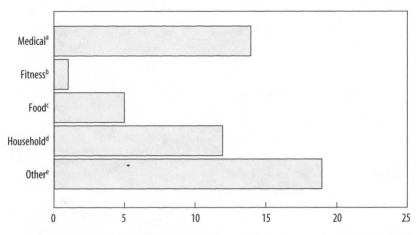

Source: Authors' compilation.

a. *AmbienCR* by Sanofi-Aventis; *Topamax* by Ortho-McNeil; Neurologics; *Boniva* by Roche Laboratories; *Mirapex* by Boehringer Ingelheim Pharmaceuticals; *Namenda* by Forest Laboratories; Abbott Laboratories; *Seroquel* by AstraZeneca; *Gemzar* by Eli Lilly Company; *Lipitor* by Pfizer; Sonafi Aventis; American Cancer Society; *Plavix* by Sanofi-Synthelabo; Bausch and Lomb.

b. The Zone Diet.

c. McDonald's Southwest salad; Organic Valley Family of Farms; Medifast; Dunkin Donuts; Eukanuba pet food.

d. *Bounce* by Proctor and Gamble; Cingular Wireless; Ebay Motors; Ann Taylor LOFT; Philips Electronics; Blockbuster; Sleepy's the Mattress Professionals; Netflix; Circuit City; Evenflo; Best Buy; Microsoft Office System.

e. Select Comfort; GameTrap by Turner Broadcasting; Crucial Technology of Micron Technology; Embassy Suites Hotels; Ask.com; MSN live search by Microsoft; Classmates.com; Hilton Hotels; Starwood Hotels and Resorts; Dish Network; Phonack; University of Phoenix; Thermage; Sprint Nextel; Elvis Presley Enterprises; Verizon; Allstate Motor Club; Vacations to Go; Comfort Suites by Choice Hotels.

As shown in figure 2-3, the nonprofit Mayo Clinic site featured far fewer ads than its commercial counterparts. Overall, there were sixteen spots, such as those for Zetia by Merck/Schering-Plough Pharmaceuticals, Lyrica by Pfizer, and Lipitor by Pfizer.

In general, these results demonstrate that nonprofit websites rely on ad revenue, although not to the same extent as their commercial counterparts. Nonprofit sites are far less likely to feature commercial advertisements or to have the real or perceived conflicts of interest that are of concern to consumers. Unsuspecting people may visit commercial sites not realizing what the sponsor's financial interests in the site are, and they may not understand how some of the information on the sites may be affected by those interests. That exposes them to either real or potential conflicts of interest in the site's provision of medical information.

FIGURE 2-3. Mayo Clinic Ads

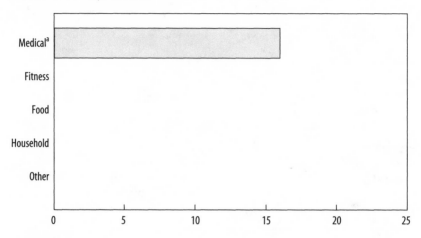

Source: Authors' compilation.

a. *Zetia* by Merck/Schering-Plough Pharmaceuticals; *Lexapro* by Forest Pharmaceuticals; *Nexium* by AstraZeneca; *Vytorin* by Merck/Schering-Plough Pharmaceuticals; *Lyrica* by Pfizer; *Lipitor* by Pfizer; *Remicade* by Centocor; *Valtrex* by GlaxoSmithKline; *Exubera* by Pfizer; *Nuelasta* by Amgen; *Abilify* by Bristol-Meyers Squibb; *Boniva* by Roche Laboratories; *Crestor* by AstraZeneca; *Rituxan* by Genentech; *Viagra* by Pfizer; *Celebrex* by Pfizer.

QUALITY OF MEDICAL INFORMATION

It is difficult to gauge the quality of medical information found on health care sites. Many state health department websites have no detailed information on specific illnesses. For commercial sites, there is little consensus on what constitutes accurate, unbiased, complete, and comprehensive advice. As patients often discover when they seek second opinions, reasonable observers may disagree on disease diagnosis and treatment.

Nevertheless, some researchers have questioned the reliability and accuracy of online information.[31] A study by Eysenbach and others demonstrates that medical websites vary enormously in the validity of their information.[32] Although the amount of accessible information has risen dramatically, there are few standards governing the provision of online materials. Some information is incomplete or inaccurate or is sponsored by pharmaceutical firms with a financial stake in particular treatments.

One way of comparing websites is to see how they handle the same illnesses. If all sites feature the same information presented essentially the same way, it suggests that everyone is drawing on the same health resources and making a good faith effort to bring accurate material to the attention of the general public. However, if there are significant differences, it raises the possibility that regardless of what independent experts might think, sites may have attempted to influence either the content or presentation of the information. That could reflect corporate interests, differences in niche strategies, or the amount of effort put into the presentation.

To look at discussions of diagnosis and treatment, we compared how the websites of WebMD.com, About.com, and MayoClinic.org handled three common diseases: breast cancer, strokes, and kidney stones. In general, the Mayo Clinic's material on each of the three was the most detailed and informative. The relative lack of advertisements and product links made Mayo's information easy to read and follow. Mayo allowed users to click "print this section" or "print all sections" when viewing information on a particular condition, so that users could obtain a paper copy of all the information that they wanted.

In contrast, WebMD had several sponsored resources on the individual disease pages, often financed by drug companies or hospitals that make a product or provide a service dealing with that condition, such as AstraZeneca for breast cancer. That poses real or potential conflicts of interest that may affect medical patients. Meanwhile, About.com had sponsored links and "health offers" all over its pages about individual diseases, making it hard to find relevant information about a disease itself. The site even included a sponsored link to material on WebMD. For example, advice on strokes included links to WebMD entitled "Get Expert Info on Strokes: Causes, Symptoms, Treatment, and Prevention." Furthermore, there were links to Healthfair.com ("Stroke Prevention: Carotid Artery Ultrasound Test. Schedule a Screening Online Today!") and HealthSmarts.com ("Stroke Facts: New Treatment Information and the Latest News on Stroke. Free Tips!").

While the Mayo Clinic provided all of its own researched information, WebMD obtained its information from a variety of sources, which usually were listed at the bottom of each page. About.com often did not identify any sources and in some cases used laypersons as "experts." That violates the Health on the Net Foundation's principle that states that quality websites should provide only information from medical professionals who are authorities in a relevant field.[33] In its section concerning breast cancer, About.com listed Pamela Stephan as its health care expert. She has no obvious medical credentials; she is instead a breast cancer survivor described as "a professional graphic designer, with a solid background in print and electronic media. She currently runs her own web design business, and volunteers for a breast cancer organization. In her spare time, she loves to cook, to grow herbs and vegetables, experiment with Origami, and stay fit." The contrasts across the three sites in information presentation and sources of information suggest there are substantial differences in the quality of the medical expertise behind each set of recommendations.

CONCLUSION

To summarize, it is apparent from this study of online content and sponsorship that there are many differences in the online content of government, commercial, and nonprofit health sites. Commercial web pages are more likely to have ads, create real or perceived conflicts of interest, and have weak disclosure of site sponsors. They also are less likely to be accessible to those with physical impairments. Public sector sites, in contrast, are more accessible and have relatively few ads, clear sponsorship, and few real or perceived conflicts of interest. Nonprofit sites are closer to the commercial model, featuring ads and sponsored links.

The advertising and sponsorship differences are troubling because they expose consumers to conflicts of interest without giving them much of a way to evaluate patient risk. Little detailed information is offered on sponsors of commercial sites, and product placements are interspersed throughout sections offering medical advice. It is hard for visitors to distinguish "expert" recommendations from those of commercial advertisers. That compromises the ability of health care providers to use online information sources to serve the interests of ordinary people.

In addition, the differences in accessibility are problematic. According to recent amendments to the U.S. Rehabilitation Act, government agencies and commercial and nonprofit entities are required to provide equal access to citizens regardless of physical impairment. Courts and policymakers have interpreted this to apply not just to bricks and mortar government but to electronic government. Part of the hope is that all citizens will share equally in the benefits of digital technology. Experts have defined universal usability as a vital goal of new technology. According to one authority, technology should enable "more than 90 percent of all households [to be] successful users of information and communications services."[34]

Based on that standard, health websites have a long way to go. Regardless of whether one looks at accessibility linked to literacy, physical impairment, or language skills, many health websites need to make much better progress than they have to date. The level at which information is written represents a major barrier to access, as does the failure of many sites to enable disabled individuals or those who do not speak English to access the information that they present online.

Software now exists that converts information to audio, text, or other kinds of electronic signals for those with visual, hearing, and physical impairments, allowing them to comprehend the contents of a website. However, sites must be designed in a way that allows the software to function properly. For example, images need "alt" text labels that identify the nature of the picture and data tables must be set up in a clear and hierarchical manner.

National data reveal that "Internet access by people with disabilities [in the United States] is one-half that of people without disabilities."[35] Only 22 percent of disabled but 42 percent of nondisabled individuals have access to the Internet. Along with disparities based on literacy and language skills, this more general digital divide raises serious issues of equity and fairness in access to public e-health resources. Unless all Americans share in the benefits of new technology, the advantages of the Internet in terms of information and service availability will be denied to those unable to take advantage of online resources.

The gap between information haves and have-nots should be a major concern to those who make health care policy.[36] Inaccessible websites hurt the underprivileged and make it difficult to justify the investment in technology that has taken place around the country. Unless these concerns are addressed, e-health will remain the domain of highly educated and affluent individuals who speak English and do not suffer from physical impairments.

CHAPTER THREE

Use of Technology

The use of technology in the United States is making progress, but it is not progressing at a rate that is transformative. For example, health care professionals are starting to rely on digital resources: half of U.S. physicians use personal digital assistants, while only 14 percent of the general population does so.[1] However, when asked in a national survey about other digital communications, only 27 percent of 1,837 responding physicians involved in direct patient care of adults said that they had adopted electronic medical records. Twenty-eight percent used e-mail to communicate with colleagues, but only 7 percent did so routinely; similarly, while 17 percent used e-mail to communicate with patients, only 3 percent did so routinely. Few also prescribed or ordered tests electronically (27 percent), received electronic alerts about potential problems when prescribing drugs (12 percent), or practiced in high-tech office settings that made regular use of electronic tools (24 percent).[2]

Other studies have shown similar slowness in the adoption of information technology by primary care physicians. Of the 2,145 doctors queried in one study, 20 to 25 percent indicated that they employed "electronic medical records, e-prescribing, point-of-care decision support tools, and electronic communication with patients." Around one-third of those questioned reported that they had no interest in any of those digital applications because of concerns over "costs, vendor inability to deliver acceptable products, and concerns about privacy and confidentiality."[3]

In this chapter, we add a consumer component to the analysis of technology use. We employ a national public opinion survey to compare the extent to which health care consumers seek medical information through face-to-face, telephone, or digital communication. Generally, we find that the revolution in health information technology still is in its infancy among ordinary consumers and health professionals alike. Although some people are making use of the Internet for health care information, digital technologies are not supplanting more traditional forms of patient contact and communication. The paucity of e-health use has negative ramifications for the future of digital medicine.

It is important to understand how extensively the public uses information technology because what consumers think and how they act has ramifications for how the revolution in health information technology unfolds. To what extent do people use digital and conventional modes to communicate with providers, acquire health care information, or make online purchases of prescription drugs and other items? To what degree is digital technology used in addition to rather than in place of conventional means of communication? The way in which people rely on new communication channels matters greatly for the future of digital medicine.

CONSUMER BEHAVIOR AND A DIGITAL REVOLUTION

One prerequisite for any digital revolution is substantial public use of a new technology. It was fifty years before the telephone was in broad use in the United States, and thirty years passed before 50 percent of the population had a television. With regard to the Internet, however, the 50 percent mark was passed less than a decade after its invention, and the same is true with regard to mobile phones.[4] Clearly, technology use occurs at a much more rapid rate now than in previous decades.

But that does not mean that health information technology has produced a revolution in the behavior of consumers or health care providers. It is impossible to proclaim a revolution in health care communications unless clinicians and consumers actually are making use of new technologies and doing so in large numbers. It does not matter how sophisticated new devices are or how much money health care providers invest in information technology. Unless people draw on such resources and see them as improving their ability to obtain quality and affordable health care, there will be few major changes in the system as a whole.

There are two aspects of consumer behavior that need to be explored. First is overall usage of health care technology. How use of digital medicine compares with use of conventional medicine is an empirical question. It is important to measure not just how many people are e-mailing their doctors but whether that number exceeds the number of those who visit doctors for face-to-face consultations or call them with questions. A number of past studies have been limited by failure to compare usage across a range of communication options.

Second is the issue of substitution versus complementarity. When people e-mail health care providers, are they doing so as a substitute for conventional communication or are they seeing old and new technologies as complementary? Our hypothesis is that more often than not, digital communication serves to complement rather than substitute for traditional forms of communication. It is most likely that individuals who employ any one technology—whether conventional or digital—will be significantly more likely to employ others. For example, it stands to reason that people visit doctors and then take information obtained through their personal encounters to surf the web for additional material. That suggests that personal or telephone encounters and use of the World Wide Web for health-related purposes are mutually reinforcing.[5]

There is little doubt that digital technologies are transforming many areas of human endeavor, from commerce and entertainment to government and communications. But as argued previously, a variety of political, social, and economic factors have limited usage levels. Low usage along with inequities based on age, gender, education, income, and geographic location suggests the importance of understanding the consumer's perspective on digital technology. The way in which change unfolds depends in part on how the public currently feels about digital medicine.

NATIONAL E-HEALTH SURVEY

To gauge the extent to which residents rely on different communication devices, we undertook a national public opinion survey regarding electronic health (see appendix A for information on sampling and questions). We asked respondents how often in the past year they had visited, called, or e-mailed a physician or other health care professional; visited a health-related website; or ordered prescription drugs or medical equipment online. A total of ten questions was asked.

Specific questions quizzed people on how often they had visited an emergency room, telephoned a doctor or other health care provider for medical or treatment advice, used e-mail to communicate with a doctor or other health care provider, used e-mail or the Internet to communicate with other people who had similar health conditions, used e-mail or the Internet to purchase a prescription drug, used e-mail or the Internet to purchase medical equipment or devices, looked on commercial Internet websites for information about health care, looked on nonprofit Internet websites for information about health care, or visited government health department websites for information about health care.

Specific response categories for each of the items included "not at all," "once every few months," "once a month," and "once a week." Because of the lack of variation on the three digital mechanisms analyzed—comparatively few reported monthly or weekly e-mails, website visits, or online purchases—we coded our outcome variables dichotomously, indicating those who did and did not engage in each of five major health communication behaviors during the previous year: making a personal visit, making phone calls, using e-mail, using the web, and making online purchases. These behaviors reflect common old and new modes of communication with health care providers.

For our analyses, we developed three category variables describing conventional communication behavior—in-person visits and telephone calls. They indicate whether a respondent had visited or called a physician or other health care professional during the previous year or did so "every few months or less" or "once a month or more." Finally, we developed a two-category variable indicating whether respondents were high or low users of digital communication technology—that is, whether they used e-mail, visited websites, or made online purchases. "Low users" include those reporting use of one digital communication method only; "high users" include those reporting use of two or more methods.

We investigate differences in usage by relying on Ronald Andersen's behavioral model of health services. The Andersen model posits that an individual's use of health services is a function of predisposing, enabling, and need characteristics.[6] According to this model, need is the most proximate cause of health service use. We conceptualize need by asking respondents to rate their current health as "very poor," "poor," "fair," "good," "very good," or "excellent." Self-rated health status is widely used in national and other surveys to identify those with the greatest health care needs, and it has been shown to be highly correlated with mortality and other outcomes. It is a way to control for health events that would lead someone to seek medical assistance.[7]

Enabling characteristics include personal/family and community resources that are thought to have an effect on usage. We operationalize personal and family resources by using insurance status (uninsured or insured) and income (0–$15,000, $15,001–$30,000, $30,001–$50,000, $50,001–$75,000, $75,001–$100,000, $100,001–$150,000, and $150,001 or more) and community resources by using geographic residence (rural or urban/suburban).

Predisposing characteristics include a variety of factors related to demographics, social structure, and health beliefs. Demographic factors are measured by using biological traits such as age (18–24, 25–34, 35–44, 45–54, 55–64, 65–74, 75–84, and 85 years or older) and gender. Social structure is operationalized by using education (0–8 years, some high school, high school graduate, some college, college graduate, or post-graduate work) in addition to race/ethnicity (non-Hispanic white, African American, Hispanic, Asian American, or something else). We collapse race/ethnicity into two categories, white and non-white.

Health beliefs include self-reported views concerning health and illness; attitudes toward health care cost, quality, and access; and knowledge about health and health care. To measure respondents' feelings concerning health and illness, we relied on three questions commonly used to measure lifestyle behaviors: how often people smoke, eat a balanced diet, and exercise. In doing so, we employed a five-point scale ranging from less to greater frequency ("not at all," "once every few months," "once a month," "once a week," and "once a day"); "every meal" and "several times a day" were added for balanced diet and smoking, respectively. Due to a lack of variation in responses, smoking was coded as a dichotomous variable for our purposes.

To measure respondents' knowledge about health and health care, we relied on three survey items developed to gauge health literacy, or "the degree to which individuals have the capacity to obtain, process, and understand basic health information and services needed to make appropriate health decisions."[8] Specific questions include how often people have someone help them read medical materials, how confident they are in filling out medical forms by themselves, and how often they have problems learning about their medical condition because of difficulty in understanding written material.[9] Response categories for these items ran from "always" and "often" to "sometimes," "occasionally," and "never."

Data analysis was used to examine the consistency of the three health literacy items. Lacking confidence in filling out forms, requiring help in reading materials, and having difficulty understanding written information were positively related to the attitudes, discussed below, that we were studying. Consequently, we used the average of these items to create the overall health literacy index used.

To study respondents' attitudes toward health services, we relied on nine items from the short-form Patient Satisfaction Questionnaire, which includes questions regarding health care affordability, access, and quality.[10] As with health literacy, principal components analysis was used to examine the consistency of the nine items as indicators of respondents' attitudes. As expected, results revealed three distinct factors reflecting affordability, access, and quality. The first factor was measured by two questions about affordability: worry about affording health care ("very worried," "somewhat worried," or "not very worried") and problems paying medical bills ("yes or "no"). The second factor was measured by two questions about access: difficulty getting appointments and ability to obtain medical care whenever needed. The third factor was measured by five questions about quality, including respondents' beliefs about whether doctors hurried too much, provided complete care, made correct diagnoses, were careful to check everything, and acted too businesslike or impersonal.

Questions about health care access and quality were measured by using a five-point scale, with responses ranging from "strongly agree" to "strongly disagree." We used the average of the individual items measuring respondents' attitudes toward access and quality to create the overall indices for those concepts. We did the same to generate the overall index for affordability. Because the two items are measured by different scales, we standardized them around their means before taking the average. Drawing on these factors, we compare consumers' use of conventional and digital medical technologies in several areas.

CONVENTIONAL VERSUS DIGITAL MEDICINE

Our analysis identified the percentage of respondents engaging in each conventional and digital health care communication mode during the previous year, including in-person, telephone, and e-mail communication; website visits; and online purchases. For ease of interpretation, we collapsed response categories on several variables in performing the analyses, including those describing respondent attitudes, lifestyle behaviors, age, education, literacy, income, and health. Logistic regressions were employed to estimate relationships between each of the communication modes and the variables of interest. These models helped us describe the extent of digital communication usage and which factors were most important with respect to the variables that we were studying.

Analyzing our national survey, we found that 87.1 percent of our general population sample reported visiting a doctor or other health care provider during the previous year and 47.4 percent indicated that they had telephoned. Reliance on conventional medicine was higher than among those who noted that they made use of different kinds of digital medicine. For example, 31.1 percent reported seeking health care information online, 7.5 percent said that they had made an online purchase (6.4 purchased prescription drugs and 2.0 percent ordered medical equipment or devices), and 4.6 percent used e-mail to communicate with a physician or other caregiver.

Our numbers are comparable to those reported by other researchers. For example, a study undertaken by Baker and colleagues regarding use of health information technology found that 6 percent of respondents indicated that they had used e-mail to contact a physician or other health care professional, while 5 percent said that they had used the Internet to purchase prescription drugs.[11] Indeed, far greater numbers of people rely on conventional than digital medicine. For all the financial resources put into new information systems and efforts by public officials to encourage use of health information technology as a way to save money, relatively few consumers are availing themselves of the new communication options. People are more comfortable with old fashioned face-to-face contact or telephone encounters than virtual or online communications. Unless usage levels rise far higher than they currently are, it is clear that policymakers will not save the billions of dollars that they are projecting through use of digital medicine.

SUBSTITUTION VERSUS COMPLEMENTARITY

Another important question concerning new technology is whether people substitute new forms of communication for more traditional forms or whether they use both forms to complement each other. The results of our national survey showed that few respondents reported using two or more digital technologies. Seventy-nine percent of digital communication

TABLE 3-1. Relationship between Types of Health-Related Communications
Percent of users

	Personal visit	Phone call	E-mail message	Website visit	Online purchase	High user
Personal visit						
No		15.7	0.0	22.1	2.8	4.3
Yes		52.8	5.2	33.9	8.3	22.7
Probability		.000***	.015*	.016*	.042*	.039*
Phone call						
No	80.4		3.0	25.3	5.6	16.7
Yes	96.1		6.4	41.3	9.8	24.3
Probability	.000*		.014*	.000***	.016*	.107
E-mail message						
No	87.6	47.2		31.2	6.8	13.6
Yes	100.0	66.7		66.7	23.3	71.8
Probability	.015*	.014*		.000***	.000***	.000***
Website visit						
No	86.3	41.7	2.2		2.9	7.1
Yes	91.9	59.8	9.0		15.5	22.3
Probability	.016*	.000***	.000***		.000****	.061†
Online purchase						
No	87.4	47.2	3.9	29.4		7.6
Yes	95.7	62.3	14.5	72.1		75.4
Probability	.042*	.016*	.000***	.000***		.000***
High user						
No	90.8	56.6	4.5	89.4	6.1	
Yes	98.5	67.7	43.1	96.9	70.8	
Probability	.039*	.107	.000***	.061†	.000***	

Source: National Public Opinion E-Health Survey, November 5–10, 2005.
***$p < .001$; **$p < .01$; *$p < .05$; †$p < .10$.

users reported using one technology only, 19 percent reported using two technologies, and 2 percent reported using three. Of single technology users, most (89.4 percent) visited health websites; relatively few e-mailed (6.1 percent) or purchased prescription drugs or medical equipment online (4.5 percent).

To illustrate substitution effects, we present data in table 3-1 from a cross-tabulation of medical communication technologies. Overall, results indicate that individuals who employed any one of the health communication strategies examined were more likely to employ the others. Respondents who visited health websites, for example, were more likely to make online purchases or call, e-mail, or visit providers in person.[12]

TABLE 3-2. Relationship between Digital and Conventional Health-Related Communications

Percent of users

	E-mail message	Website visit	Online purchase	High user
Personal visit				
None	0.0	22.1	2.8	4.3
Every few months	4.7	35.2	7.0	18.1
Once a month or more	6.8	29.9	11.8	37.9
Probability	.023*	.022*	.011*	.000***
Phone call				
None	3.0	25.3	5.6	16.7
Every few months	6.2	42.6	9.3	23.0
Once a month or more	7.4	35.5	12.3	29.0
Probability	.043*	.000***	.035*	.212

Source: National Public Opinion E-Health Survey, November 5–10, 2005.
***$p < .001$; **$p < .01$; *$p < .05$.

Respondents who visited health websites were more likely to use it for e-mailing and online purchases than individuals who communicated in person or over the telephone. Sixty-six percent of e-mailers and nearly 75 percent of online purchasers visited health information websites, and 33.9 percent of in-person and 41.3 percent of telephone communicators did so, demonstrating the complementary nature of digital medicine for many consumers.

Our survey results show that all respondents who relied on e-mail also reported in-person visits. But the reverse also was true. Respondents who made in-person visits were much more likely to telephone or e-mail physicians and to make online purchases. That suggests strong support for the complementarity hypothesis. Consumers who make use of one technology are more likely to draw on other kinds of technologies.

The relationship between the rate of digital and the frequency of conventional communication usage is further explored in table 3-2. The frequency of conventional communications such as personal office visits or phone calls is broken down into categories of "not used," "used every few months," or "used once a month or more." In general, our survey results indicate that the rate of digital communication use increases with an increase in the frequency of engaging in conventional communication behavior. That is true with regard to e-mail and online purchases in particular; with those items, the percentage of consumers saying that they used each technology increases progressively along with an increase in frequency from no visits or telephone calls to visiting or calling "every few months" or "once a month."

Those reporting no in-person visits or telephone calls were also least likely to visit health websites, although those reporting visiting or calling "every few months or less" were more likely to report visiting health websites than those reporting doing so "once a month." That again demonstrates the extent to which old and new communication uses complement one another.

EXPLANATIONS OF HEALTH TECHNOLOGY USAGE

To this point, we have explored public usage patterns at the bivariate level. However, it is important to examine those patterns at the multivariate level in order to control for a number of different factors. Table 3-3 reports results from logistic regression models predicting use of each of the five health communication modes during the previous year. We control for a variety of factors thought to influence health care behavior, such as age, gender, race, income, place of residence, and education. We also included public perceptions about a variety of lifestyle behaviors; attitudes toward health care cost, access, and quality; and factors such as health status, having health insurance, and literacy, all of which are thought to have a link to individuals' health care orientation.

Overall, the models fit the data very well. None of the independent variables were highly correlated with one another, and tolerance tests showed no problematic multicollinearity. Covariates representative of at least two Andersen model elements proved significant to each of the five communication modes analyzed.

Predisposing Factors: Although age was not significantly related to four of the five communication modes studied, results indicate that older individuals were significantly less likely to seek health care information online than younger individuals. While women were neither more nor less likely to e-mail providers or make online purchases, they were twice as likely to visit in person or make a telephone call and 73 percent more likely to seek health information online. Better educated respondents were also more likely to make telephone calls, visit websites, and make online purchases. No significant associations could be identified between educational level and e-mail use and in-person visits or between race and any of the five communication modes analyzed.

TABLE 3-3. Logistic Regression of Types of Health-Related Communications and Select Variables[a]

Variable	Personal visit	Phone call	E-mail message	Website visit	Online purchase
Age	.104 (.069)	−.010 (.045)	−.077 (.110)	−.199 (.053)***	−.021 (.098)
Female	.718 (.224)**	.620 (.149)***	.106 (.348)	.550 (.170)**	.012 (.274)
Minority	−.270 (.282)	.151 (.200)	.404 (.431)	−.110 (.226)	.009 (.375)
Education	−.008 (.107)	.143 (.070)*	.083 (.157)	.444 (.082)***	.330 (.131)*
Perception of costs	−.003 (0.154)	.189 (.101)†	.115 (.233)	.228 (.115)*	.374 (.183)*
Perception of accessibility	0.157 (0.144)	.031 (.087)	.083 (.200)	.174 (.095)†	.138 (.153)
Perception of quality	−.297 (.190)	.029 (.110)	−.219 (.251)	−.014 (.124)	.144 (.198)
Exercise	.061 (.078)	.109 (.050)*	−.007 (.116)	.002 (.057)	.028 (.096)
Balanced diet	.012 (.079)	.074 (.053)	.480 (.181)**	.039 (.061)	−.109 (.092)
Smoking	−.162 (.272)	−.078 (.189)	−.818 (.624)	.054 (.209)	−.264 (.387)
Health literacy	−.158 (.150)	−.233 (.096)*	−.169 (.198)	.137 (.113)	−.099 (.181)
Income	0.150 (0.88)†	.097 (.060)	.191 (.134)	.182 (.064)**	.296 (.102)**
Health insurance	1.11 (.303)***	.538 (.157)*	.254 (.612)	.081 (.269)	−.068 (.461)
Urban residence	.147 (.249)	−.053 (.157)	1.13 (.510)*	.323 (.176)†	.551 (.334)†
Self-perceived health	−.430 (.113)***	−.312 (.070)***	−.438 (.151)**	−.088 (.077)	−.120 (.124)
Constant	2.24 (1.26)†	−1.023 (.820)	−4.79 (2.08)*	−4.24 (.966)***	−4.69 (1.60)**
Pseudo R^2	.148	.106	.128	.213	.121
N	917	910	923	883	920

Source: National Public Opinion E-Health Survey, November 5–10, 2005.
a. Table reports logistic regression coefficients with the standard errors in parentheses.
***$p < .001$; **$p < .01$; *$p < .05$; †$p < .10$.

Findings indicate that individuals with more negative attitudes toward health care costs were more likely to visit health websites, make online purchases, and telephone a physician or other provider. Similarly, individuals with more negative perceptions of accessibility were more likely to look for health information online. Whereas individuals with stronger health literacy were less likely to telephone a health care provider, those reporting more frequent exercise and healthy eating habits were more likely to telephone and e-mail, respectively. Other combinations of respondent attitudes and medical communication use failed to yield significant findings.

Enabling Factors: Respondents with higher incomes were more likely than those with lower incomes to contact health care providers in person but not by e-mail or telephone. They also were more likely to visit health websites and make online purchases. Whereas respondents with health insurance were three times more likely than those without to report visiting a health care provider in person and nearly three-quarters more likely to do so over the telephone, they were neither more nor less likely to e-mail, visit health websites, or make online purchases. That is in contrast to individuals living in urban/suburban neighborhoods, who were more than three times more likely than rural residents to e-mail providers, nearly three-quarters more likely to make online purchases, and one-third more likely to visit health websites; however, they were neither more nor less likely to telephone or see a provider in person.

Need: Our results reveal an inverse association between better perceived health and each of the communication modes examined in the study. However, only the relationships between better perceived health and e-mail, telephone use, and in-person visits achieved statistical significance. In addition, respondents employing multiple digital technologies (high users) were more likely to report in-person visits or telephone calls than those employing one (low users). Finally, we examined differences between high and low users of digital technology. High users were somewhat more likely to visit health websites than low users, and they were much more likely to e-mail providers or make online purchases. Thus, whereas most single technology users visited health websites, most high users visited websites and added e-mail or online purchases to their digital communications arsenal. The percentage of multiple technology users increased along with higher frequency of conventional communication behavior.

Only five of the fifteen respondent characteristics examined proved significantly related to multiple digital technology use. Both bivariate and multivariate results indicate that better educated individuals with poorer health status living in urban/suburban areas were more likely to be high users than less educated individuals with better health status living in rural areas. They also indicate that individuals with stronger health literacy tended to eschew use of multiple technologies, relying more often on one technology. Multivariate results reveal a positive association between the reported frequency of exercising and multiple usage as well.

Interestingly, there was not much of a digital divide between high and low users of digital communications (see table 3-4). Neither income level nor age mattered. Educational differences were significant, but only at the .10 level, indicating a modest association. That suggests that other factors are far more crucial in explaining the variation in technology use.

TABLE 3-4. Logistic Regression of Select Variables on High Use
of Digital Communications[a]

Variable	High use
Age	−.046 (.108)
Female	.004 (.320)
Non-white	−.020 (.411)
Education	.253 (.142)†
Perception of costs	.048 (.212)
Perception of accessibility	.246 (.178)
Perception of quality	−.075 (.234)
Exercise	.184 (.108)†
Balanced diet	.056 (.119)
Smoking	−.579 (.468)
Health literacy	−.377 (.221)†
Income	.014 (0.73)
Health insurance	−.420 (.505)
Urban residence	.741 (.418)†
Self-perceived health	−.497 (.146)***
Constant	−.002 (1.971)
Pseudo R^2	.153
N	311

Source: National Public Opinion E-Health Survey, November 5–10, 2005.

a. Table reports logistic regression coefficients, with standard errors in parentheses. High use (use of two or three technologies) is compared with low use (use of one technology).

***$p < .001$; **$p < .01$; *$p < .05$; †$p < .10$.

CONCLUSION

Our analysis indicates that the e-health revolution remains in a very early stage. Few people are using many of the digital tools, and usage is going to have to rise dramatically in order to reap the desired benefits of the technology revolution. As a sign of the slow pace of technology adoption in the e-health arena, we found a much higher percentage of respondents reporting conventional in-person and telephone contact with health care personnel (87.1 and 47.4 percent, respectively) than e-mail contact (4.6 percent), website visits (31.1 percent), or online purchases (7.5 percent). For most new forms of communication, usage remains at negligible levels.

Our results demonstrate that more attention needs to be devoted to boosting overall use of health technology. Relatively few individuals (7.1 percent) report use of two or more digital technologies during the previous year. At 87.1 percent, our figure for in-person contact approximates that from the National Health Interview Survey (NHIS), which reports that 82 percent of adults 18 years of age and older had an office visit with a doctor or other health care professional in 2004.[13] Although we did not find a relationship between in-person visits and education, our study reflects NHIS findings that individuals visiting a physician or other health professional were more likely to be older, female, white, higher income, and insured.

Our figure for website usage, 31.1 percent, also approximates the figures from other national surveys, including those from the Pew Internet and American Life Project (30 to 38 percent), Brodie and others (31 percent), and Ybarra and Suman (41 percent).[14] It also approximates the figure from Dickerson and others (33 percent), a survey of 315 patients at three urban primary care clinics and one of the few non-nationally representative samples we could identify.[15] Only the May-June 2004 Pew survey reports the percentage of American adults using the Internet to purchase prescription drugs (4 percent), although Baker and others reports the percentage of Internet users having done so (5 percent).[16]

With respect to e-mail, Baker and others reports that only 6 percent of Internet health users had e-mailed a physician or other health care provider, and the December 2002 Pew survey reports that just 7 percent of e-mail users had exchanged e-mails with a doctor or other health professional.[17] The relatively low percentage of respondents in our survey who reported e-mailing providers (4.6 percent) or purchasing prescription drugs (6.4 percent) does not differ substantially from what was reported a few years earlier in those surveys.

Together, these results indicate that the online revolution is developing at a snail's pace, far below the rate desired by policymakers. More often than not, one communication form serves to complement rather than substitute for other forms. That is reflected in the finding that individuals who employed any one technology—whether conventional or digital—were significantly more likely to employ the other options as well. The three Internet-based technologies were especially correlated: few respondents e-mailed providers or made online purchases without also searching for health information online. Indeed, virtually all users of a single digital technology visited health care websites, whereas most users of multiple technologies combined website visits with online purchases or e-mail use. That implies that use of the World Wide Web for health-related purposes may be mutually reinforcing, with health information searches typically serving as the foundation on which more interactive forays into the health care Internet are built.

Although digital technologies typically complement rather than substitute for conventional communication, there is evidence that some substitution is taking place. Whereas no respondents reported using e-mail unless they had also seen a physician or other provider in person and only 2.8 percent made an online purchase without having in-person contact, a little more than one-fifth (22.1 percent) searched for health information online although they did not report an in-person consultation during the previous year.

Not only were respondents' visits to health websites more likely to be independent of their conventional health system contacts, respondents also were more likely to visit websites as the frequency of conventional contact declined. That suggests that website visits may serve as substitutes for conventional contact at least part of the time. These findings are in stark contrast to the findings for e-mail and online purchases, which correlated more strongly with in-person contact. It may be that those correlations are more contingent on provider cooperation—that is, whether providers make e-mail available to patients or write the prescriptions necessary to allow them to purchase drugs online.

In general, our research findings indicate that efforts to promote usage need to focus on specific populations. Women coordinate health services, both for themselves and their families. They also suffer from greater morbidity and poorer health than men.[18] It should not be surprising, therefore, that we found a positive relationship between being female and engaging in both conventional and digital health-seeking behavior. That is also reflected in previous studies, which indicate not only that women are more likely to visit a physician or other health care professional than men but also that they are more likely to visit health care websites.[19] Respondents in poorer health were more likely to e-mail their physicians or other health care providers, as was the case for their in-person and telephone contacts, again reinforcing findings from earlier work.[20]

Although we failed to detect significant relationships between respondents' health beliefs and in-person medical encounters, we did identify associations between respondents' attitudes toward health care costs and lifestyle and other forms of medical communication. Moreover, those with more negative cost experiences were more likely to telephone, visit websites, and make online purchases. Not only do these findings support the expectation that individuals who are more attuned to their health are more likely to contact providers outside of regular office visits, they also support the expectation that individuals with greater difficulty affording care are more likely to seek alternative sources of health information, advice, and supplies on the World Wide Web. As did results of other studies, our results indicate that respondents who sought health information over the Internet tended to be younger than those who did not, whereas those visiting health care professionals in person tended to be older, at least according to our bivariate results.[21]

Especially worrisome are inequities based on education, income, and area of residence. Even after controlling for other factors, poorly educated, rural respondents with lower incomes were less likely to report visiting health websites or making online purchases than better educated, urban respondents with higher incomes. Whereas rural respondents were also less likely to use e-mail, poorly educated health information technology users living in rural areas were less likely to make use of multiple digital communication modes as well. The conclusion that better educated individuals are more likely to search for health information online is perhaps the most consistent finding across multivariate studies of health-related Internet use to date.[22] There also is evidence that the effects of respondents' characteristics may vary across racial and ethnic groups.[23] That insurance coverage predicted conventional but not digital communication behavior implies that while being uninsured poses a barrier to more traditional forms of health service usage, it does not pose a barrier to Internet access and that uninsured individuals are just as likely as insured individuals to go online for health-related purposes.

Our findings suggest that e-mail use in digital medicine may be a hybrid, driven by health status (as with conventional health system contact) and also by urban/rural location (as with website visits and online purchases). Like other forms of digital communication, e-mail requires access to the underlying telecommunications infrastructure, which is more developed in urban and suburban than rural areas: whereas 39 percent of Americans living in urban or suburban neighborhoods have high-speed Internet access, only 24 percent of rural Americans do.[24] Unlike website visits, however, e-mail use is contingent on prior access to physicians and other health care professionals and therefore may be dependent on factors that drive use of the conventional health system, such as health status and the extent of insurance coverage.

Although online purchases may be contingent on prior access to physicians and other health care professionals, our results indicate that prior contact may be an absolute prerequisite for e-mail use. Thus, whereas some respondents made online purchases without being in personal contact with a health care provider, no respondents used e-mail without also being in personal contact with a health care provider. That being the case, health status may be a more important driver of e-mail use than the purchase of prescription drugs or medical equipment online.

It is clear that there are highly salient sociodemographic barriers to increased use of health information technology, including impediments arising primarily from the preferences and concerns of providers and patients and the ways that they interact with one another.[25] Especially salient to providers are financial concerns associated with reimbursement, long-term funding, and other costs.[26] For example, while lack of payment for e-mail consultations may not be a problem for providers who are paid a fixed amount per patient no matter how many services they render, e-mail–specific reimbursement may be necessary to stimulate further investment in health information technology by providers paid on a fee-for-service basis.[27]

There also are nonfinancial costs that limit providers' enthusiasm for new technologies, including time, staff, and other resources devoted to learning new systems and staying up-to-date on changes in hardware and software. Evidence suggests that there may be workload increases if new technologies complement rather than substitute for office visits.[28] Health care providers have to devote more time to patients if office visits are going to stimulate e-mailing and other types of digital contact.

Lack of standardization and the piecemeal development of the telecommunications infrastructure in health care is another important obstacle.[29] Right now, many health care providers have digital systems that do not interface with those of other professionals. That complicates communication between caregivers and also between patients and doctors and makes it difficult to improve communication.

Finally, there are several sociolegal barriers to widespread acceptance of health information technology, including patient concerns about privacy and security and changes in the that way e-health affects relationships among patients, providers, and the organizations with which they interact. If doctors and patients communicate electronically and online records detail a person's entire medical history, can consumers be guaranteed that those electronic records will be safe and secure? It is clear that government officials must work harder on a variety of fronts if they wish to see the increases in productivity, efficiency, and access to health benefits expected with expanded use of the World Wide Web in health care.

CHAPTER FOUR

Relationship between Use of Digital Technology and Attitudes toward Health Care

Digital materials affect how people make decisions regarding their health and medical care. For example, Baker and others found in a national public opinion survey that one-third of respondents using the Internet for health purposes claimed that such electronic resources had positively influenced their health care choices. In particular, respondents stated that digital medicine altered the way that they ate, exercised, or managed their health care needs and that it improved their general understanding of medical symptoms, conditions, and treatments.[1]

However, analysts remain divided over the relationship between individuals' use of electronic health resources and their assessment of the health care system in general. David Blumenthal of Massachusetts General Hospital, for example, worries that patient satisfaction with the quality of medical care will decline in a wired world.[2] In his view, the professional autonomy that doctors currently have is threatened by an environment in which consumers get medical information directly online. He worries that if patients can get health consultations and order prescriptions drugs independently of their personal physicians, the quality of medical care will be undermined.

Other observers dispute that pessimistic interpretation, arguing that digital medicine actually will improve the quality of health care. For example, Newt Gingrich believes that information technology is the key to improving care while reducing overall costs. He suggests that technology gives people greater control over their health care and allows patients to learn more about their medical options.[3] Hillary Clinton and Barack Obama made similar arguments when they introduced their plans for health care during the campaign for the Democratic Party's presidential nomination. Both claimed in their respective proposals that health information technology would improve care while saving billions of dollars a year in federal spending.[4]

At this early stage in the online medical revolution, what is needed are national public opinion data that measure whether digital technology helps people feel better about the health care that they receive personally from their doctors. Is technology associated with improved consumer knowledge, higher health literacy, or positive perceptions about the quality and cost of health care?[5] Does use of digital medical resources lead to viewing the health care system positively or believing that health care is more affordable and of higher quality?

Technology advocates expect that use of health information technology will be positively associated with improved consumer health behaviors and attitudes. Indeed, that assumption is at the heart of many recent proposals regarding health information technology. Advocates believe that adoption of digital communications will make people feel more positive regarding access, affordability, and quality of the system as a whole. For example, widespread adoption of electronic medical records is expected to cut costs, reduce errors, and improve patient satisfaction with health care.

But whether digital technology actually is associated with improvements in consumers' views on health care is an empirical matter.[6] It is not enough simply to assert an association in order to sell specific policy proposals; there must be concrete evidence to support the claim. Unless there is a strong link between use of digital technologies and improvement in public attitudes, it will be difficult for electronic health policy advocates to attract the needed public investments or to transform the health care system.

In this chapter, we use our national public opinion survey to determine the relationship between technology usage and attitudes toward the health care system. We asked a series of questions regarding participants' satisfaction with medical care, knowledge level, experiences with costs, and views about the health care system to see whether any relationship exists between technology usage and how consumers assess the quality of physician care. Is there any association between the type of information technology—conventional or digital—used and worries about the cost of medical care or how respondents rate the performance of the health care system?

Our survey allowed us to examine eighty different possible associations between how people get medical information (in person, over the telephone, or from digital sources) and their satisfaction with health care quality, worries about cost and access, lifestyle choices, health status, and health literacy. We sought to determine whether use of digital health care technology is associated with greater patient satisfaction, lower costs, higher-quality service, and improved access to care, as claimed by information technology proponents.

After undertaking our analysis of national survey data, we find that only 6 percent of the associations were significant in the direction desired by policymakers; by that, we mean that consumers who relied on various digital resources also felt positively about health care quality, access, and affordability. Given those results, we argue that the revolution in health care technology is not yet associated with positive attitudes toward the U.S. health care system. Few people are using digital technology to get information, other than by visiting health care websites, or to communicate with medical personnel. Moreover, there are few favorable associations between usage and how they feel about the cost or quality of health care in the United States.

In the long run, public perceptions about health care quality, access, and affordability are the key to greater use of health information technology. What people think affects what they do. There is nothing in the e-health revolution so far that guarantees that usage will rise or be associated with positive attitudes toward the health care system. As we point out in the conclusion to this book, policymakers must undertake a variety of new initiatives to realize the benefits of digital medicine.

HEALTH ATTITUDES AND HEALTH BEHAVIOR

The relationship between health attitudes and behavior is complex. People sometimes say one thing and do another. They may perceive things in a particular manner, but that does not mean that their perceptions always govern their behavior. They may be misinformed, unaware, ambivalent, or confused, and any one of those states could produce a gap between attitude and action.

In addition, even if attitudes and behavior match up perfectly, there is no guarantee that policy will achieve the desired outcomes for the system as a whole. Those outcomes rest on features beyond consumer attitudes and behavior. The long-term impact of particular communications technologies ultimately depends on economic investment, political decisions, institutional settings, and social structures, among other things.

Those points notwithstanding, it is important to look at the link between attitudes and behaviors because attitudes affect behavior and behavior influences attitudes. Sorting out causal links requires attention to the nature of the relationship between attitudes and behaviors. Researchers must be sensitive to various conceptions of causality, especially in regard to health policy.

In this analysis, we investigate the relationship between respondents' use of technology and attitudes about the health care system. Our goal is to determine whether use of in-person, telephone, and especially digital communication—such as by visiting health websites, e-mailing doctors, and making medical purchases online—is associated with positive perceptions about health care. We analyze the data to see whether there is any relationship between use of communications technology and respondents' self-perceived health status, lifestyle choices, health literacy, and views on health care quality, affordability, and access.

We control for a variety of factors, such as age, gender, race, income, education, place of residence, having health insurance, party identification, and ideology, all of which are thought to affect individuals' views about the health care system. Demographic forces are important in health care because of well-documented differences in care linked to age, race, gender, income, education, and place of residence. As noted earlier in this volume, people experience health care in different ways and empirical analysis must control for the differences.

In addition, political characteristics such as party identification and ideology influence views on health care. Republicans and conservatives are more likely than Democrats and liberals to favor market solutions to health care. By contrast, Democrats see the government as playing an important role in health care—for example, by facilitating access for needy people or helping those who cannot afford their own quality health care.

Finally, perceived health status and having health insurance are important variables. Those in poor health are more likely to visit doctors and seek medical assistance, so it is crucial to control for how healthy an individual is. In addition, those who have health insurance tend to be better educated and have higher incomes than those who do not. Individuals without health insurance experience problems of affordability, access, and quality of care; one therefore would expect their attitudes to differ from the attitudes of those with health insurance.

We recognize that correlation does not equal causality and that a positive association between use of digital technology and favorable perceptions of the affordability and quality of care does not guarantee either actual cost savings or quality medical care. Nevertheless, we argue that consumer perceptions are important to debates over electronic health. If citizens do not believe health information technology is improving their health care or making medicine more affordable, they are going to be far less interested in making use of digital medicine or investing tax dollars in promoting it. Convincing ordinary people that technology will improve quality of care and save money in the process is the best way to increase technology usage and decrease public expenditures. Unfavorable public perceptions of digital medicine make it very difficult for health care reformers to accomplish either goal.[7]

HEALTH STATUS AND CONSUMER LIFESTYLES

We start our analysis of the relationship between technology use and attitudes toward health care by looking at health status and consumer lifestyle. As noted earlier, our health status question asks people to rate their current health as excellent, very good, good, fair, poor, or very poor. We regress different means of communication on that item, controlling for standard factors such as age, education, gender, race, ethnicity, family income, political party affiliation, and ideology. Those variables allow us to hold constant factors thought to influence a variety of health perceptions.

Table 4-1 presents the regression results, and as one would expect, seeing oneself in good health is associated with being younger, better educated, richer, and making few in-person visits or phone calls to doctors. There is no relationship between health status and visiting online health websites, purchasing prescription drugs or medical equipment online, or e-mailing doctors.

Table 4-2 presents the results for consumer lifestyles. We rely on commonly used indicators of health behavior—such as how often people smoke, eat a balanced diet, or exercise—to assess lifestyle. We measure these variables on a five-point scale running from "not at all" and "once every few months" to "once a month," "once a week," and "once a day." The results demonstrate that people who e-mail their doctors

TABLE 4-1. Logistic Regression of Select Variables on Self-Perceived Health Status[a]

Variable	Self-perceived health status
Personal visit	−.43 (.07)***
Phone call	−.19 (.07)**
E-mail message	−.02 (.15)
Website visit	−.17 (.09)
Online purchase	−.16 (.25)
Age	−.08 (.03)**
Female	.01 (.10)
Minority	−.05 (.13)
Education	.18 (.04)***
Income	.13 (.03)***
Health insurance	−.08 (.15)
Democratic party affiliation	.09 (.06)
Liberal ideology	.12 (.07)
Constant	−1.73 (.48)***
Adjusted R^2	.24
F	13.37***
N	502

Source: National Public Opinion E-Health Survey, November 5–10, 2005.
a. Table reports the unstandardized regression coefficients, with standard errors in parentheses.
***$p < .001$; **$p < .01$; *$p < .05$.

more, who are female, or who are white are more likely to say that they eat a balanced diet. There are no associations between lifestyle and visiting or calling doctors, visiting health websites, or making online purchases. There is no relationship between electronic means of communication and getting exercise, but a positive association exists between exercise and personal or phone contacts.

The only other significant variables on that item were age, self-reported health status, and income. Healthier people with higher incomes were most likely to say that they exercised frequently. There were associations with smoking for visiting doctors, ideology, age, and education. Those who visited doctors infrequently or who were politically conservative, older, or well educated were the least likely to say that they smoked.

AFFORDABILITY AND ACCESSIBILITY

We also examined the association between medical communications and perceptions about the affordability and accessibility of health care. We

TABLE 4-2. Logistic Regression of Select Variables on Lifestyle Choices[a]

Variable	I eat a balanced diet	I exercise	I do not smoke
Personal visit	.12 (.10)	.23 (.11)*	−.21 (.13)*
Phone call	.00 (.09)	.21 (.10)*	.03 (.12)
E-mail message	.38 (.19)*	.08 (.21)	.10 (.26)
Website visit	−.134(.12)	.07 (.13)	−.02 (.11)
Online purchase	−.06 (.32)	.02 (.35)	−.09 (.26)
Age	.05 (.04)	−.04 (.04)	.16 (.05)**
Female	.51 (.13)***	.09 (.14)	.20 (.17)
Minority	−.36 (.17)*	−.17 (.19)	.19 (.25)
Self-perceived health	.05 (.06)	.40 (.06)***	.14 (.08)
Education	.10 (.06)	.00 (.06)	.26 (.08)***
Income	.06 (.04)	.04 (.05)*	.04 (.06)
Health insurance	.20 (.19)	−.03 (.21)	−.30 (.27)
Democratic Party affiliation	−.03 (.08)	−.04 (.09)	.09 (.12)
Liberal ideology	−.05 (.09)	−.13 (.09)	−.26 (.13)*
Constant	3.07 (.63)***	4.13 (.69)***	2.91 (.91)***
Adjusted R^2	.05	.10	.06
F	2.88***	4.82***	3.11***
N	495	496	501

Source: National Public Opinion E-Health Survey, November 5–10, 2005.
a. Table reports unstandardized regression coefficients, with standard errors in parentheses.
***$p < .001$; **$p < .01$; *$p < .05$.

looked at several different measures: how worried respondents were about whether they could afford the health care needed by their family ("very worried," "somewhat worried," or "not very worried"); whether they or a family member had had any problems paying medical bills in the past year ("yes" or "no"); and whether they agreed that those who provide medical care sometimes hurry too much , whether they agreed that it is hard to get an appointment for medical care right away, and whether they agreed that they are able to get medical care whenever they need it. The possible responses for the last three items were "strongly agree," "agree," "uncertain," "disagree," or "strongly disagree."

Table 4-3 presents regression results for these items. The major significant variables for worry about the affordability of health care included visiting health sites, age, and income; those who visited websites frequently, were younger, and were poor were most likely to express worry. Those who phoned their doctor often, visited health websites frequently, were younger, or were poor had the most difficulty paying their medical bills.

TABLE 4-3. Logistic Regression of Select Variables on Perceptions of Affordability and Accessibility[a]

Variable	I worry about the affordability of health care		I have problems paying medical bills		I believe medical care is to hurried		I find it hard to get an appointment		I am not able to get medical care when needed	
Personal visit	.11	(.06)*	−.00	(.03)	−.13	(.09)	−.07	(.09)	−.00	(.07)
Phone call	.01	(.05)	.07	(.03)*	.12	(.08)	.10	(.08)	.05	(.07)
E-mail message	−.02	(.11)	−.03	(.06)	−.43	(.18)*	−.18	(.17)	−.19	(.14)
Website visit	.03	(.07)*	.07	(.04)[*]	.24	(.11)*	.10	(.11)	.04	(.09)
Online purchase	.30	(.18)	.13	(.10)	.48	(.30)	.52	(.29)	.37	(.24)
Age	−.05	(.02)*	−.04	(.01)***	−.07	(.04)*	−.12	(.04)***	−.08	(.03)**
Female	.25	(.07)*	−.01	(.04)	−.00	(.12)	.07	(.11)	−.01	(.10)
Minority	−.17	(.10)	−.01	(.05)*	−.11	(.16)	.28	(.15)	.01	(.13)
Self-perceived health	−.11	(.03)**	−.05	(.02)**	−.01	(.05)	−.05	(.05)	−.02	(.4)
Education	.02	(.03)	−.00	(.02)	−.09	(.05)	.00	(.05)	−.02	(.04)
Income	−.14	(.02)***	−.04	(.01)***	−.01	(.04)	.06	(.04)	−.00	(.03)
Health insurance	.70	(.11)***	.18	(.06)***	.57	(.18)***	.51	(.17)**	.42	(.14)**
Democratic Party affiliation	.04	(.05)	.04	(.02)	.07	(.07)	−.01	(.07)	.05	(.06)
Liberal ideology	.03	(.05)	−.06	(.03)	.09	(.08)	.02	(.08)	−.01	(.07)
Constant	−3.71	(.36)***	−1.97	(.19)***	−3.52	(.58)***	−4.62	(.57)***	1.63	(.37)***
Adjusted R^2	.20		.13		.06		.06		.02	
F	8.53***		6.06***		3.27***		3.30***		1.79*	
N	497		497		497		495		497	

Source: National Public Opinion E-Health Survey, November 5–10, 2005.
a. Table reports unstandardized regression coefficients, with standard errors in parentheses.
***$p < .001$; **$p < .01$; *$p < .05$.

In addition, we found that the category of those who feel that medical personnel who provide medical care sometimes hurry too much is associated with e-mailing doctors infrequently, visiting health websites, having insurance, and being young. Young respondents also were most likely to report that it was hard to get an appointment for medical care right away. By contrast, elderly individuals were most likely to feel that they were able to get medical care when they needed it.

HEALTH LITERACY

Three survey items are commonly employed to gauge health care literacy: how often people have someone help them read medical materials, how confident they are in filling out medical forms by themselves, and how often they have problems learning about their medical condition

TABLE 4-4. Regression of Medical Communications Technology and Select Variables on Health Literacy[a]

Variable	I need help reading medical materials	I am not confident in filling out medical forms	I have problems understanding written information
Personal visit	.01 (.07)	.07 (.08)	.08 (.07)
Phone call	.15 (.06)*	.10 (.08)	.09 (.07)
E-mail message	.32 (.13)*	.13 (.16)	−.07 (.14)
Website visit	−.08 (.08)	−.17 (.10)	−.06 (.09)
Online purchase	.24 (.22)	.59 (.27)*	.36 (.24)
Age	.03 (.03)	.06 (.03)	.03 (.03)
Female	−.18 (.09)*	−.06 (.10)	.06 (.10)
Minority	.09 (.12)	.09 (.14)	.04 (.13)
Self-perceived health	−.06 (.04)	−.09 (.05)	−.04 (.04)
Education	−.09 (.04)*	−.14 (.05)**	−.13 (.04)**
Income	−.02 (.03)	−.05 (.04)	−.05 (.03)
Health insurance	.14 (.13)	.31 (.16)	.26 (.14)
Democratic Party affiliation	−.00 (.06)	.05 (.07)	.00 (.06)
Liberal ideology	.04 (.06)	.05 (.07)	.07 (.07)
Constant	−5.22 (.44)***	.55 (.52)	−5.10 (.37)***
Adjusted R^2	.07 .11	.07	
F	3.67***	5.47***	3.57***
N	496 495	496	

Source: National Public Opinion E-Health Survey, November 5–10, 2005.
a. Table reports unstandardized regression coefficients, with standard errors in parentheses.
***$p < .001$; **$p < .01$; *$p < .05$.

because of difficulty understanding written material (possible responses were "always," "often," "sometimes," "occasionally," or "never"). We use these items to investigate respondents' use of technology and their feelings about digital medicine.

Table 4-4 examines the relationship between types of medical communication and health literacy. Those who phone and e-mail doctors frequently, who are male, or who are poorly educated were most likely to say that they need help reading medical materials. The only avenue of communication that had a significant link to confidence in filling out forms was online purchasing. Those who made medical purchases online were more likely to feel unconfident about completing forms. Well-educated individuals were most likely to indicate that they were not confident about filling out forms. Education was associated with respondents' having problems learning about their medical condition because of difficulty understanding written information: those who were poorly educated were most likely to say that they had problems.

QUALITY OF HEALTH CARE

The quality of health care is a dominant topic of broader discussions about the U.S. health system. Many health care reforms are designed to improve medical quality and make sure that patients are satisfied with their health care experience. Not only is high consumer satisfaction seen as a desirable end in itself, high-quality medical experiences represent a way to boost public support for the system as a whole and convince taxpayers that investments in this area will be beneficial.

To gauge how medical communications relate to views about quality of care, we examine four indicators: whether respondents agree that their doctor's office has everything needed to provide complete medical care, that their doctors provide correct diagnoses, that doctors are careful to check out everything when examining and treating them, and that doctors act too businesslike and impersonal toward them. Answers were given on a five-point scale, from "strongly agree" to "agree," "uncertain," "disagree," or "strongly disagree."

Table 4-5 presents regressions for the relationship between respondents' use of medical communications technology and other variables and their perceptions about the quality of health care. Believing that doctors provide complete medical care is significantly associated with visiting or e-mailing doctors frequently and being politically conservative. People who phone their doctor infrequently and who are older are most likely to feel that doctors diagnose health conditions correctly. Individuals with better perceived health are more likely to feel that doctors check everything during examination and treatment. There is an association between thinking that doctors are not too business-like and impersonal and visiting doctors frequently and being well educated. These results suggest some favorable associations for the quality of health care and use of digital communications.

CONCLUSION

To summarize, we did not find consistent benefits of information technology for a number of consumer perceptions about health care. As Blumenthal has warned, there are no guarantees that a wired world is going

TABLE 4-5. Regression of Medical Communications Technology and Select Variables on Perceptions of Quality of Health Care[a]

Variable	Doctors do not provide complete medical care	Doctors make me wonder whether their diagnoses are correct	Doctors do not check everything when treating me	Doctors are too businesslike and impersonal
Personal visit	−.19 (.07)**	−.05 (.08)	−.13 (.08)	−.23 (.09)**
Phone call	.05 (.07)	.16 (.08)*	.09 (.07)	−.06 (.08)
E-mail message	−.31 (.14)*	−.05 (.16)	−.06 (.15)	.05 (.17)
Website visit	.05 (.09)	.01 (.10)	.06 (.09)	.13 (.10)
Online purchase	.15 (.23)	.50 (.27)	.20 (.25)	.53 (.28)
Age	.03 (.03)	−.08 (.03)**	−.01 (.03)	−.05 (.03)
Female	−.02 (.09)	−.05 (.11)	−.05 (.10)	−.17 (.11)
Minority	−.12 (.13)	.02 (.14)	−.08 (.14)	−.15 (.15)
Self-perceived health	−.04 (.04)	−.08 (.05)	−.09 (.05)*	−.09 (.05)
Education	.03 (.04)	−.01 (.05)	−.04 (.05)	−.13 (.05)**
Income	−.03 (.04)	−.03 (.04)	.04 (.04)	−.00 (.04)
Health insurance	.04 (.04)	.23 (.16)	.50 (.15)**	.07 (.16)
Democratic Party affiliation	.11 (.06)	.04 (.07)	.03 (.06)	.08 (.07)
Liberal ideology	.13 (.06)*	.14 (.07)	.06 (.07)	.08 (.08)
Constant	1.88 (.45)***	−3.47 (.52)***	1.55 (.39)**	−2.91 (.55)***
Adjusted R^2	.04	.04	.02	.04
F	2.62***	2.55**	1.78*	2.47**
N	496	495	491	500

Source: National Public Opinion E-Health Survey, November 5–10, 2005.
a. Table reports unstandardized regression coefficients, with standard errors in parentheses.
***$p < .001$; **$p < .01$; *$p < .05$.

to produce positive attitudes toward the health care system.[8] People's perceptions of health care quality, access, or affordability do not necessarily become more positive because they communicate with medical professionals electronically instead of in person.

In this study, we examine eighty possible links between medical communications and perceptions about health care quality, affordability, and access; literacy; and health status. As shown in table 4-6, 76 percent of the overall relationships between in-person, telephone, e-mail, and digital communications and health care evaluations were nonsignificant, meaning that few benefits were associated with the use of each communications approach. And of the associations that were statistically significant, 15 percent were in an undesirable direction, meaning that they were associated with worse outcomes with respect to perceptions of the health care system. Only 9 percent were in the desired direction from the

TABLE 4-6. Summary of Substantive Associations between Conventional and Digital Health-Related Communications

Percent

	Overall	Conventional	Digital
Nonsignificant	76 (61/80)	66 (21/32)	84 (40/48)
Desirable	9 (7/80)	12 (4/32)	6 (3/48)
Undesirable	15 (12/80)	22 (7/32)	10 (5/48)
N	80	32	48

Source: National Public Opinion E-Health Survey, November 5–10, 2005.

standpoint of the health system as a whole. The paucity of positive results gives pause to those who envision dramatic positive changes in public attitudes following the implementation of health information technology.

The relationship was nonsignificant between attitudes toward health care and sixty-six percent of uses of conventional (personal visits or phone calls) and 84 percent of uses of digital medical communications (e-mail use, website visits, or online purchases); the relationship was in the desired direction for 12 percent of uses of conventional and 6 percent of uses of digital communications; and the relationship was in an undesirable direction for 22 percent of uses of conventional and 10 percent of uses of digital communications.

Table 4-7 breaks those substantive results down in greater detail. The table shows whether there was a desirable significant (+), undesirable significant (-), or nonsignificant (0) substantive association with the preferred health outcome, such as good health, healthy lifestyle, affordable and accessible health care, health literacy, and quality care, after controlling for a variety of sociodemographic characteristics.

Ten of the sixteen regressions show no significant relationship between frequency of visiting doctors and desirable health outcomes. Of the remaining six relationships, three are in the desired direction (meaning that they show a positive relationship between seeing doctors more frequently and having good outcomes) and three in an undesirable direction (meaning that seeing doctors frequently is associated with undesirable outcomes). For example, those who report frequent visits to doctors also are likely to say that they have poor health, smoke, and worry over the affordability of health care. In addition, those with more frequent doctor visits are more likely to get exercise, to believe that doctors provide

TABLE 4-7. Summary of Substantive Associations between Health-Related Communications and Views of Health Care and Select Variables[a]

Variable	Personal visit	Phone call	E-mail message	Health-related website	Online purchase
Better health status	–	–	0	0	0
Lifestyle					
I eat a balanced diet	0	0	+	0	0
I exercise	+	+	0	0	0
I do not smoke	–	0	0	0	0
Affordability/accessibility					
I do not worry over affordability	–	0	0	–	0
I have no problem paying bills	0	–	0	–	0
Medical care is not hurried	0	0	+	–	0
It is not hard to get an appointment	0	0	0	0	0
I am able to get care when needed	0	0	0	0	0
Health literacy					
I do not need help reading	0	–	–	0	0
I am confident filling out forms	0	0	0	0	–
I have no problem understanding information	0	0	0	0	0
Quality					
Doctors provide complete medical care	+	0	+	0	0
Doctors make correct diagnoses	0	–	0	0	0
Doctors check everything	0	0	0	0	0
Doctors are not too businesslike	+	0	0	0	0

Source: National Public Opinion E-Health Survey, November 5–10, 2005.

a. A minus sign indicates an undesirable association with an outcome variable; a plus sign indicates a desirable association; and a zero reveals no significant relationship, controlling for other factors.

complete care during office visits, and to believe doctors are not too businesslike in their approach.

There are eleven nonsignificant, one desirable, and four undesirable associations for telephone calls to doctors. On the desirable side, making frequent phone calls to health providers was associated with getting exercise. On the undesirable side, making frequent phone calls to physicians was associated with poor health status, problems paying medical bills, needing help with reading materials, and wondering whether doctors reach the correct diagnosis.

Twelve of the sixteen associations with e-mail use were nonsignificant, indicating no relationship between frequency of e-mailing doctors and most of the outcomes studied. Of the other four relationships, three were in the desired direction and one was not. For example, there was a relationship between the frequency of e-mailing physicians and having a balanced diet, thinking medical care was not hurried, and believing that doctors provide complete care. However, e-mailing doctors often was also associated with needing help reading medical materials.

Thirteen of the sixteen relationships for visits to health websites were nonsignificant and three were significant but undesirable: worrying about health care affordability, having problems paying medical bills, and feeling that medical care is hurried were negatively associated with frequent website visits.

There were nonsignificant associations for online medical purchases for fifteen of the sixteen health care outcomes and one undesirable association. No matter how often medical patients purchased medications or health equipment online, there were no positive outcomes in terms of perceived health status, lifestyle choices, or views about affordability, access, or quality of health care. The only exception came in regard to the health literacy item of filling out medical forms: individuals who were most likely to purchase medical goods online were least likely to feel confident about medical documents in general.

At this point, the e-health revolution remains more hope than reality. Large numbers of people do not use digital or electronic technology to deal with medical professionals.[9] There is a significant digital divide in the areas of gender, age, education, and income. Those who are older, male, or less educated or who have low incomes make less use of some communication tools than do their counterparts. That limits the ability of technology to make a positive difference in people's health.[10]

Positive associations between using digital technology and having desirable perceptions of health care quality, affordability, and accessibility were evident for only 6 percent of respondents. E-mailing health providers was the use of digital communications most likely to have a positive association. That was reflected in the finding regarding balanced diet and the belief that medical care was complete and unhurried. In our analysis, there were few positive associations between use of digital technology and perceptions of health care quality or affordability.

However, research by other scholars has found a relationship between use of electronic health resources and positive ties to the health care system. For example, those who reported having the most connections to the health care system were also likely to make the most extensive use of digital resources and to feel good about the experience. They were more likely to seek prescription renewals over the Internet, make use of online consultations, and make appointments online.[11]

But the overall lack of strong associations in our study demonstrates that government officials need to work harder on several fronts if they wish to generate positive benefits in health care. As discussed later in this volume, technology usage levels must rise considerably above current levels and individuals must have positive experiences that make them feel better about their health care.[12] Unless many more people e-mail doctors, visit websites, or purchase drugs or medical equipment online and feel good about the results, the ability to achieve positive gains through information technology will be limited. Raising usage levels is a prerequisite to securing the gains of digital medicine for health consumers.

CHAPTER FIVE

Digital Disparities

Eliminating disparities in health care in the United States has been a national priority for a number of years.[1] Inequality is a problem with regard to race and ethnicity in particular. Because of the country's history of slavery and discrimination, it has been difficult to produce equality of opportunity or results. People of different backgrounds experience varying degrees of access and present clear contrasts in health care quality and outcomes.

Gaps in mortality and disease rates persist across income and racial lines. There are well-known economic and racial disparities in infant deaths, cardiovascular disease, and age-adjusted death rates for diabetes.[2] For example, the average life expectancy is 77.7 years for whites and 72.2 years for blacks.[3] Those differences in health and longevity have endured for a long period of time, suggesting that race remains a deep and enduring division in the United States.

One recent study of Medicare reimbursements found extensive variation in medical treatment by race and locale. For example, the researchers discovered that in some states there was "a difference of 12 percentage points between the white rate and the black rate" for patients receiving mammograms. Similarly, African Americans suffering from diabetes "were less likely than whites to receive annual hemoglobin testing." In several southern states, the rate for leg amputations among African Americans was double the rate for whites.[4]

Others have discovered discernible differences by race and ethnicity among people lacking health insurance. A Kaiser Family Foundation research project found that 36 percent of Hispanics had no health insurance; the corresponding figure was 33 percent for Native Americans, 22 percent for African Americans, 17 percent for Asian Americans, and 13 percent for non-Hispanic whites. Overall, two-thirds of those without insurance were poor.[5]

Despite the obvious implications of such disparities, only a handful of studies have examined the relationship between race, ethnicity, and health website usage.[6] Three studies have found a significant association between race/ethnicity and going online for health-related purposes. However, two of the studies (Dickerson and others and Hsu and others) were not nationally representative.[7] The other (Ybarra and Suman) neglected to include income as a predictor.[8] The last study is problematic because available evidence indicates that racial and ethnic differences disappear after controlling for income and socioeconomic status.

In this chapter, using data from our national public opinion survey, we examine variations in use of health websites by respondents' education, income, race, and ethnicity. We find that important demographic differences remain in access to health information technology. Policymakers need to address those differences if they want to close the digital divide and bring the benefits of electronic health care to all Americans.

DEMOGRAPHIC DISPARITIES

Between 2000 and 2004, the number of Americans going online to search for health information nearly doubled, from 50 to 95 million.[9] That spurt in digital activity reflects the increasing popularity of the Internet, efforts by various organizations to improve its accessibility, and reductions in the cost of computing. People understand that there is a tremendous amount of information online, and they are taking advantage of new communication features.

Although consumers' ability to acquire information over the Internet has increased, disparities in access to digital technology compromise the ability of some populations to benefit fully from electronic resources.[10] For example, there are well-documented gaps in use of information technology based on education, age, income, and geographic location. Those who are younger and better educated, who have more money, and who live in urban and suburban areas are most likely to use the Internet. Individuals with lower incomes and less education who live in rural areas are least likely to rely on websites or other forms of digital communication.[11] Sometimes that is due to lack of wiring or inadequate broadband access; other times it is linked to lack of money to pay for computers or digital access.

Even more troubling are indications of a gap based on race and ethnicity. One recent national survey of general Internet use, for example, found that while 70 percent of whites go online, only 57 percent of African Americans do;[12] another study found that 65 percent of whites go online but only 37 percent of Hispanics.[13] Those results are problematic because they indicate that Hispanics and African Americans are less likely to make use of technology and therefore are less able to take advantage of online medical material.

As telecommunications technology becomes further integrated into health service provision, such gaps in access to information reinforce existing inequities. To the extent that government agencies want consumers to rely on digital medicine in order to improve service delivery and reduce costs, it is important to understand how access differs among different racial and ethnic groups. If racial differences are present in regard to electronic health care services, they undermine the equity and justice of the U.S. health care system; they also compromise the ability of policymakers to achieve the full benefits of digital medicine.

Several factors contribute to racial differences in use of both health care services and information technology.[14] One problem is unequal access to quality health care.[15] Individuals from different socioeconomic backgrounds do not have the same opportunities for effective and affordable care. Those who are older and come from impoverished backgrounds, for example, are less likely to receive various kinds of medical care. They also do not see the need for or value of digital communications and so generally are not part of the technology revolution. They do not understand how the Internet can enrich their lives.

There is growing concern over how the digital divide creates inequities in the use of online resources.[16] Age is a major characteristic distinguishing users from nonusers. While older people are less likely to use the Internet, the same is true for those of limited education and income. Individuals who are poorly educated or who lack financial resources do not access digital information and are not able to surf the net for electronic health care.[17]

Finally, there are significant racial differences in literacy levels. The National Assessment of Adult Literacy found that on a scale from 0 (low literacy) to 500 (high literacy), the average score for whites (288) was higher than that for Asian Americans (271), African Americans (243), and Hispanics (216).[18] Those differences mean that Hispanics have the greatest difficulty in comprehending reading material and therefore in understanding online medical resources. Website developers must take that finding into consideration when they design their sites.

Given the increasing use of the Internet to provide remote monitoring and other health-related services, it is important to investigate what types of inequalities exist in health website usage. To what extent are race, ethnicity, income, education, age, and gender linked to usage of digital medical resources? If we can identify specific disparities, it will help public officials improve the ways in which they provide access for different types of patients.

ANALYSIS OF MEDICAL WEBSITE USAGE BY RACE AND ETHNICITY

To investigate demographic disparities, we examined health website usage by racial and ethnic background. Among the 828 respondents to our national public opinion survey who reported race or ethnicity there were 670 non-Hispanic whites (80.9 percent), 58 African Americans (7.0 percent), 54 Hispanics (6.5 percent), and 46 Asian Americans or individuals in some other category (5.6 percent). Although the percentage of respondents identifying as African American, Hispanic, and Asian American/Other in the general population (12.1, 13.6, and 7.5 percent, respectively) exceed the percentage included in our poll, that is not unusual for projects that attempt to contact hard-to-reach populations.[19]

We focus more on African Americans and Hispanics than Asian Americans because historically African Americans and Hispanics have suffered greater deprivation in access to information. Asians Americans are not a great concern with respect to the digital divide in particular because they tend to rely on digital technology to an even greater extent than non-Hispanic whites.[20] Indeed, that tendency was borne out in our survey. Of respondents who reported searching for health information online during the previous year, 43.5 percent belonged to the Asian American/Other category, 33.7 percent were white, 31 percent were African American, and 20.4 percent were Hispanic. We emphasize web usage in this study because it is the most prevalent use of digital medicine.[21] Those who e-mail

Table 5-1. Variation in Website Use by Race and Ethnicity
Percent of users

	White	African American	Hispanic	Asian American/ Other
Age				
Less than 65 years	40.5	36.4	21.6	50.0
65 Years	14.9	0.0	0.0	0.0
Probability	.000***	.010**	.625	.043**
Gender				
Male	27.0	18.8	21.7	31.6
Female	38.1	35.7	19.4	51.9
Probability	.003***	.177	.546	.144
Education				
High school or less	16.3	16.7	8.8	30.8
Some college/college degree	44.3	46.4	40.0	51.6
Probability	.000***	.015**	.009***	.175
Health literacy				
Poor to fair	18.8	37.5	0.0	57.1
Good to excellent	35.8	31.3	23.8	47.1
Probability	.003***	.508	.115	.471
Income				
Less than $30,000	20.0	27.3	13.0	26.7
$30,000 or more	43.3	35.0	38.1	70.0
Probability	.000***	.418	.058	.013**
Self-perceived health				
Very poor to fair	25.9	16.7	27.3	33.3
Good to excellent	35.8	34.8	18.6	47.1
Probability	.030**	.198	.396	.316
N	670	58	54	46

Source: National Public Opinion E-Health Survey, November 5–10, 2005.
***$p < .01$; **$p < .05$; *$p < .10$.

physicians or purchase medicine or health care equipment online are far less numerous than those who search the Internet for medical information.

A variety of factors other than race and ethnicity affect web usage. For example, other researchers have found that features such as self-perceived health status, income, education, age, gender, and health literacy are relevant for patient attitudes and behaviors.[22] Generally, people's orientation with respect to health care is affected by their health, age, and gender, among other considerations.

Table 5-1 breaks down web usage for various racial groups by these factors. Generally, we found that 14.9 percent of whites age 65 or above

Table 5-2. Logistic Regression of Website Usage by Racial and Ethnic Group and Select Variables[a]

Variable	White	African American	Hispanic	Asian American/ Other
Age	−0.24 (0.06)***	−0.16 (0.16)	0.19 (0.32)	−0.35 (0.23)
Female	0.21 (0.14)	0.82 (0.82)	−0.52 (1.01)	0.89 (0.76)
Education	0.50 (0.08)***	1.10 (0.39)***	1.44 (0.57)**	0.56 (0.29)**
Health literacy	0.16 (0.13)	−0.69 (0.53)	1.86 (1.01)*	−0.69 (0.50)
Income	0.01 (0.04)	−0.00 (0.12)	−0.24 (0.22)	−0.06 (0.14)
Self-perceived health	−0.14 (0.08)*	0.30 (0.31)	−1.01 (0.59)*	0.27 (0.34)
Constant	−2.24 (0.74)***	−4.24 (2.89)	−9.12 (5.16)*	−1.02 (2.35)
Pseudo R^2	0.157	0.334	0.483	0.276
N	670	58	54	46

Source: National Public Opinion E-Health Survey, November 5–10, 2005.
a. This table reports logistic regression coefficients, with standard errors in parentheses.
***$p < .01$; **$p < .05$; *$p < .10$.

reported accessing health websites but no African American, Hispanic, or Asian American/Other respondents age 65 or above indicated that they did so. Bivariate results demonstrate that better educated individuals within each group were more likely to search for health information online, though that finding was significant only for whites, African Americans, and Hispanics.

Women and persons with better self-perceived health were more likely to access health-related websites within the white, African American, and Asian American/Other categories; however, the associations were statistically significant only for whites. By contrast, among Hispanics, men and persons in worse self-perceived health were more likely to access online information, although neither association was statistically significant.

In general, respondents with higher incomes were more likely to visit websites, although again, results were significant for white and Asian American/Other respondents only. Whereas stronger health literacy was associated with use of websites among whites and Hispanics, it was associated with lower use among African Americans and Asian Americans/Others. But the association was statistically significant among Hispanics; no Hispanic respondents with poor to fair health literacy reported searching for health information online.

Table 5-2 reports our logistic regression analysis, the results of which indicate that the models fit the data very well. We found that older age was significantly negatively associated with use of health websites among whites, but not among other groups. By contrast, higher education was associated with greater use of health websites in all groups, although the association seemed to be stronger among African Americans and Hispanics than among whites and Asian Americans/Others.

Better perceived health was significantly negatively associated with health website use among whites and Hispanics, but there is no such evidence for African Americans or Asian Americans/Others. Stronger health literacy was significantly positively associated with health website use among Hispanics, but not among other groups. No significant associations could be identified between website usage and gender or income.

VARIATION IN OVERALL USAGE BY SOCIAL BACKGROUND

To help us understand the racial and ethnic patterns reported in our study, we examined the characteristics of respondents engaging in each form of conventional and digital health care communication. Table 5-3 shows that there were few significant associations between education, income, and residence and conventional communication behavior; social background, then, did not influence the extent to which people visited or called physicians.

However, for digital communications, respondents who were better educated, who had higher incomes, or who lived in urban/suburban areas were more likely than respondents who were less well educated, who had lower incomes, or who lived in rural areas to report e-mailing providers, visiting websites, or making online purchases. That helps to explain why Hispanics lag behind whites in use of e-health resources. They often have less education and lower incomes, and those barriers undermine their use of digital medical information.

Interestingly, though, this increase in use of digital technologies did not hold in regard to insurance status. Being insured increased the chances of visiting a provider in person or over the telephone, but it had no significant association with digital communication usage. Whereas older people were more likely to make in-person visits, they were less likely to visit health care websites; middle-aged respondents, however, were more likely to make online purchases. There is also a gender gap, with women being more likely than men to make in-person visits, place telephone calls, and visit health information websites.

TABLE 5-3. Variation in Use of Types of Health-Related Communications by Subgroup

Percent of users

Subgroup	Personal visit	Phone call	E-mail message	Website visit	Online purchase	High use
Age						
18–44	85.3	49.1	4.3	39.3	6.9	17.7
45–64	87.9	46.5	6.0	39.0	10.3	23.6
65+	93.8	50.5	3.4	33.0	2.9	15.6
Probability	.012*	.636	.344	.000***	.005**	.385
Gender						
Male	83.5	38.7	4.0	26.1	7.9	21.0
Female	91.1	54.7	4.9	37.0	7.5	20.9
Probability	.001**	.000***	.492	.001**	.803	.987
Race						
White	90.0	48.0	4.6	33.7	7.5	20.1
Non-white	83.6	48.1	6.0	31.0	7.3	22.2
Probability	.019*	.967	.425	.514	.919	.724
Education						
0–11 years	88.5	43.0	5.1	9.0	3.8	27.3
12 years	86.2	43.9	3.5	17.9	3.9	18.9
13–16 years	89.4	50.1	4.2	42.1	6.5	15.4
17+ years	89.0	52.6	8.6	53.3	18.2	31.4
Probability	.631	.228	.122	.000***	.000***	.040*
Perception of costs						
Positive	90.3	48.3	4.5	33.2	7.1	19.1
Moderate	84.2	34.9	6.2	27.7	6.2	23.8
Negative	86.1	61.3	4.2	39.7	9.6	23.8
Probability	.070	.000***	.661	.086†	.455	.628
Perception of accessibility						
Positive	90.3	49.0	4.2	29.7	5.8	16.4
Moderate	86.7	45.8	7.0	36.0	9.1	25.3
Negative	90.7	54.8	2.5	45.5	11.0	23.1
Probability	.301	.285	.112	.004**	.071	.204
Perception of quality						
Positive	91.8	48.1	5.9	30.3	4.8	16.1
Moderate	88.9	47.7	4.0	33.1	9.3	22.5
Negative	87.8	67.1	6.7	43.7	5.5	22.6
Probability	.390	.008**	.388	.105	.060†	.460

(continued)

TABLE 5-3 *(continued)*

Subgroup	Personal visit	Phone call	E-mail message	Website visit	Online purchase	High use
Exercise						
None	86.6	43.2	5.0	25.3	6.9	20.0
Occasional	88.9	49.1	4.8	38.6	8.9	20.4
Daily	87.9	49.2	4.6	31.2	6.6	20.8
Probability	.753	.402	.976	.009**	.478	.993
Balanced diet						
No meals	84.0	36.0	1.4	26.4	8.0	22.2
Occasional meals	87.0	48.2	2.4	30.2	8.9	16.4
Every meal	89.2	50.6	5.7	34.6	7.2	21.2
Probability	.344	.057†	.065†	.263	.733	.711
Smoker						
No	89.2	49.0	5.3	33.4	8.1	21.6
Yes	83.9	45.4	1.7	30.9	5.6	16.4
Probability	.053†	.389	.039*	.517	.275	.387
Health literacy						
Poor/fair	85.4	51.2	7.3	17.1	7.3	44.4
Good	86.5	54.2	8.1	22.2	8.1	38.9
Very good	94.7	57.0	2.6	30.0	7.0	18.1
Excellent	87.0	44.3	4.8	37.7	7.5	17.9
Probability	.013*	.011*	.185	.003**	.988	.044*
Income ($)						
0–30,000	83.1	47.6	3.8	20.3	2.6	18.0
30,000–75,000	88.6	46.3	3.7	39.6	10.2	21.8
75,000–100,000	92.3	56.6	6.4	49.3	7.9	16.2
100,000 or more	89.1	48.9	9.6	52.8	14.9	24.5
Probability	.104	.452	.095†	.000***	.001**	.745
Health insurance						
No	71.9	37.7	3.2	27.5	5.7	23.5
Yes	91.0	49.8	5.0	34.3	7.6	20.1
Probability	.000***	.013*	.386	.146	.458	.638
Residence						
Rural	87.4	47.9	1.7	27.7	4.4	12.2
Urban/suburban	89.1	47.8	6.0	36.3	8.9	23.6
Probability	.461	.961	.004**	.013*	.017*	.030*
Self-perceived health						
Very poor/poor	93.2	70.2	8.5	24.6	5.1	50.0
Fair	89.3	51.9	8.3	25.2	9.9	40.0
Good	93.2	51.1	3.4	31.9	6.8	16.9
Very good	87.4	41.8	4.0	38.5	8.1	17.4
Excellent	79.7	44.1	3.7	33.9	7.4	15.9
Probability	.000***	.001**	.113	.056†	.764	.002**

Source: National Public Opinion E-Health Survey, November 5–10, 2005.
***$p < .001$; ** $p < .01$; *$p < .05$; †$p < .10$.

From these data, it is apparent that those who are poor were more likely to communicate conventionally than digitally with medical professionals. Such individuals appear to be more comfortable with receiving health care through face-to-face encounters. They want the personal touch, and their health care choices reflect their sentiments. People with higher incomes and healthier life style behaviors (such as eating a balanced diet, getting exercise, and not smoking) were more likely to e-mail health care providers. These findings reinforce the racial and ethnic differences noted earlier in this chapter.

CONCLUSION

This analysis uses a national public opinion survey to determine the characteristics of various racial/ethnic groups seeking online health information. Several previous studies have identified the overall percentage of U.S. adults and/or Internet users searching for health information,[23] but only one reported the percentage of the total population seeking health information online stratified by race.[24] That study reported 1999 online data for white (34.0 percent) and African American (19.0 percent) respondents only.

By contrast, our study reports the prevalence of online searches among whites, African Americans, Hispanics, and Asian Americans/Others. If one uses the 1999 data as a baseline, the digital divide has narrowed for African Americans with respect to health care. That is good news for those concerned about racial disparities in health website usage in the United States; however, the relatively low percentage of Hispanics reporting use of health websites indicates that the ethnic divide has not disappeared.

In order to boost web use, health care providers need to communicate more clearly with Hispanic patients. Low use among Hispanics may reflect, in part, language difficulties for individuals who do not speak English; Hispanics have language barriers that most other large minority groups do not encounter. But it also is a question of trust with elderly Hispanic patients. Research by Sabogal, Scherger, and Ahmadpour argues that among Hispanic patients, "patient distrust and perceptions of physician disrespect [of Hispanic patients] are common."[25] When health care has a technological component, physician-patient miscommunication becomes more likely. For that reason, these scholars recommend better understanding of language limitations and cultural background in the provision of electronic health information.

Education may interact with cultural values to influence health Internet use. Among key Hispanic cultural values is *personalismo*, in which personal relations are of central importance and connections with individuals are preferred to connections with institutions. That is closely related to another key value, *confianza* (trust), which leads to a preference for establishing relationships of trust with individuals over extended periods of time.[26] Because of these cultural beliefs, the impersonal nature of the Internet may not be congruent with widely held Hispanic values and therefore may complicate web use among members of the community.

In a similar vein, due to a legacy of racial discrimination, African Americans have greater distrust of institutions, including the health and medical system, than other groups, which makes it difficult for them to feel comfortable accessing health resources. That is the case regardless of whether the form of communication is traditional or digital.[27] It will be hard to make much progress with digital medicine until the members of minority groups develop reasonable trust in online resources.

The fact that better educated individuals are more likely to search for health information online is reflected in several research studies.[28] Although well-educated respondents of all types were more likely to access health information in our study, the relationship was especially strong for African Americans and even stronger for Hispanics. Relative to whites with comparable education, therefore, less well educated minorities are at a greater disadvantage, suggesting that education may interact with one's life experiences and cultural expectations to influence use of the Internet for health information. Indeed, educational institutions with greater minority enrollment are less likely to provide students with Internet access.[29]

Minority access to health information is constrained because often digital material is written at a reading level that exceeds that of many minority users.[30] According to Eysenbach and his colleagues, that makes the problem of online medical advice not always being accurate, complete, or consistent even more difficult.[31] Because many minority users have a low reading level, developing complete and accurate online health resources that they can benefit from will be challenging. Poor literacy is an especially important concern in health care due to clear links between low health literacy, race/ethnicity, and inadequate understanding of medical materials.[32] That the association between health literacy and Internet use is statistically significant only for Hispanics may reflect the fact that many Hispanics face language barriers to access as well as more general constraints.

The city of New Ulm, Minnesota, is piloting a $100 million initiative known as the Center for Healthcare Innovation that seeks to improve quality of care through new technology. It aims to bring electronic medical records and new outreach efforts to a neighborhood that is one-third Hispanic, one-third African American, and one-third white. Ninety percent of the people in town get health care from the Allina Hospital and Clinic, and the hospital is undertaking a special effort to find people who are at greatest risk and treat them before they become chronic sufferers.[33]

Such efforts are important because research has shown that Internet use declines with age for all groups.[34] But while nearly 15 percent of elderly white respondents sought health information online, no elderly African American or Hispanic respondents did so. That implies that not only do African Americans and Hispanics fall disproportionately on the wrong side of the digital divide, but that being elderly further amplifies the effect of minority status on health Internet use.

Elderly minorities are less well educated and have lower incomes and more limited English proficiency than younger minorities.[35] Consequently, they are less likely to possess the skills and resources necessary to purchase a computer, use the Internet, or visit various websites. Although similar gaps in income and education exist between older and younger non-Hispanic whites, the percentage of older whites that are poor and lack a high school diploma is not nearly as high nor is the gap between age cohorts quite as wide.[36] That could explain, in part, why at least some elderly whites reported visiting a health website, in contrast to elderly African Americans and Hispanics.

From this analysis, it is clear that race and ethnicity remain a serious problem for the future of digital medicine. Those demographic characteristics interact with age, education, literacy, and income in important respects. Policymakers cannot increase use of health information technology without addressing the gaps in access that exist for some groups. It will prove difficult to gain economies of scale unless greater numbers of older, less well-off, and less educated people begin to use online resources. Only then will we begin to narrow the digital divide and attract more people to use e-health resources.

CHAPTER SIX

Information Acquisition

As documented in earlier chapters, considerable differences exist between public and private health care websites. Commercial sites are much more likely to have product ads, to be unclear about who their sponsors are, and to create real or potential conflicts of interest. In contrast, government sites rarely feature ads, clearly are noncommercial in nature, and do not present the financial conflicts of interest seen with some private sites.[1] They do not attempt to sell commercial products or push services linked to financial backers.

Those contrasts make it crucial to understand the type of people who visit different kinds of websites. Despite the promise of digital technology, there has been relatively little empirical research regarding who relies on which types of sites.[2] Are there differences between users of government and nongovernment websites? What implications do any variations have for digital medicine?

We employed our national public opinion survey data to examine the relationship between users and types of websites used. In particular, we looked at user characteristics such as age, literacy, place of residence, and attitudes toward health care services in the United States to see whether they reveal a preference for use of public or private sector sites. We sought to determine whether there are systematic differences in the visitors to the alternative sources of information.

In general, we find variations linked to age, education, and urban/rural location. Those who rely on private sites are more likely to be younger, to live in urban areas, and to be poorly educated. Websites are not neutral in whom they attract; there are discernible differences between users of the two kinds of sites.

Given those findings, we argue that it will require a concerted effort on the part of policymakers to improve the quality, accessibility, and relevance of online health care information. Important differences in patterns of use have ramifications for how society makes use of electronic resources and attempts to overcome the gap between electronic haves and have-nots. We cannot make progress in electronic health without understanding the interaction between health website content and user characteristics.

ANALYSIS OF HEALTH WEBSITE VISITORS

We asked respondents to our national survey about forms of health care communication, satisfaction with health services, health knowledge level, and lifestyle behaviors. We also asked for basic demographic information, including age, gender, race, health insurance status, education level, residence, income, and perceived health. Our goal was to identify any differences between visitors to public and commercial websites and any systematic visitation patterns.

Respondents were quizzed regarding how often in the past year they had visited a government or private website. Specific categories included "not at all," "every few months or less," "once a month," and "once or more a week." In addition to identifying the frequency with which respondents accessed each type of site, we coded each variable dichotomously, indicating those who did and did not visit a particular type of site during the previous year.

According to our responses, more than twice as many of our survey respondents visited private websites (29.6 percent) as public websites (13.2 percent). However, few reported accessing either public or private websites more than a handful of times during the course of the year. Only 23.6 percent and 18.9 percent of private and public website visitors, respectively, said that they did so at least once a month.

Both public and private website visitors were more likely than nonvisitors to be better educated and to report greater concerns about health care access. Younger individuals living in urban areas who had stronger health literacy and greater concerns about the affordability of health care were more likely to visit private but not public websites. Efforts to close the digital divide must recognize such differences in user characteristics, and relatively low usage levels require a concerted effort to improve the quality, accessibility, and relevance of Internet health information.

We looked at differences in website usage based on age, gender, attitudes, education, lifestyle, literacy, locality, income, and health (see table 6-1). It is important to analyze respondents' demographic characteristics because of their well-documented links to use of technology. Furthermore, it is crucial to look at self-perceived health status, because people who are ill should be more likely to visit public and/or private health sites. We also examine a variety of attitudes regarding health care access, affordability, and quality. Finally, we account for lifestyle (diet, exercise, and smoking) as well as whether an individual has health insurance.[3]

In general, we found a number of significant differences. Younger females with better educations, higher incomes, and more negative attitudes toward health care access were more likely to report visiting both public and private sector websites than less well educated older males with lower incomes and more positive attitudes toward access. Respondents with more negative attitudes toward health care quality also were more likely to visit both government and private websites.

These behaviors are also true of respondents with more negative attitudes toward health care affordability, although results did not achieve statistical significance. Whereas respondents with occasional or daily exercise regimes, stronger health literacy, urban/suburban residences, and better perceived health were more likely to visit private sector websites, they were neither more nor less likely to visit public ones.

No significant associations could be identified between any form of website usage and race, balanced diet, smoking, and insurance status. There was no difference in website usage between public and private sector sites.

EXPLAINING INFORMATION ACQUISITION

To this point, we have examined usage levels at the bivariate level. An obvious limit of that approach is the inability to control for a variety of demographic and social variables that are relevant to website use. We incorporate a range of characteristics in order to determine which are most important with respect to influencing individuals' use of public or private health websites.

TABLE 6-1. Variation in Use of Public and Private Sector Websites by Subgroup
Percent of users

Subgroup	Public sector site	Private sector site
Age		
18–44	13.6	37.3
45–64	18.4	35.9
65+	5.9	13.4
Probability	<.0001***	<.0001***
Gender		
Male	9.1	25.6
Female	16.2	34.2
Probability	.003**	.007**
Race		
White	13.8	32.0
Non-white	13.0	28.1
Probability	.809	.342
Education		
0–11 years	5.1	6.4
12 years	5.8	15.9
13–16 years	15.5	40.4
17+ years	28.9	50.0
Probability	<.0001***	<.0001***
Perception of costs		
Positive	14.3	30.8
Moderate	10.4	27.7
Negative	16.0	37.1
Probability	.349	.184
Perception of accessibility		
Positive	11.2	28.1
Moderate	14.6	34.9
Negative	24.3	39.8
Probability	.001***	.023*
Perception of quality		
Positive	8.9	29.1
Moderate	15.5	30.8
Negative	16.4	42.3
Probability	.027*	.098
Exercise		
None	11.9	22.6
Occasional	16.5	36.4
Daily	11.7	29.8
Probability	.128	.007**

(continued)

TABLE 6-1 (*continued*)

Subgroup	Public sector site	Private sector site
Balanced diet		
No meals	9.5	23.3
Occasional meals	12.6	28.8
Every meal	14.2	32.6
Probability	.495	.211
Smoker		
No	13.7	31.8
Yes	11.9	27.8
Probability	.513	.313
Health literacy		
Poor/fair	7.3	14.6
Good	14.9	16.7
Very good	12.9	29.0
Excellent	14.1	35.6
Probability	.643	.001***
Income		
0–30,000	8.2	19.7
30,000–75,000	14.0	37.3
75,000–100,000	19.2	47.3
>100,000	29.8	47.2
Probability	<.000***	<.001***
Health insurance		
No	11.5	25.6
Yes	14.1	32.4
Probability	.439	.136
Residence		
Rural	11.3	24.4
Urban/suburban	15.0	35.2
Probability	.137	.001***
Self-perceived health		
Very poor/poor	11.9	21.1
Fair	12.3	24.2
Good	14.8	30.2
Very good	13.5	36.4
Excellent	13.0	31.9
Probability	.952	.059

Source: National Public Opinion E-Health Survey, November 5–10, 2005.
$*p < .05; **p < .01; ***p < .001$.

TABLE 6-2. Logistic Regression Models of Website Usage and Select Variables

Variable	Public sector site		Private sector site	
Age	0.90	(0.79–1.03)	0.83***	(0.75–0.91)
Female	1.23	(0.95–1.59)	1.14	(0.89–1.47)
Non-white	0.93	(0.53–1.65)	0.85	(0.55–1.32)
Education	1.53***	(1.29–1.80)	1.57***	(1.37–1.80)
Perception of costs	1.04	(0.78–1.38)	1.25*	(1.00–1.56)
Perception of accessibility	1.28*	(1.01–1.62)	1.20†	(0.99–1.44)
Perception of quality	1.12	(0.82–1.53)	1.03	(0.80–1.32)
Exercise	0.98	(0.86–1.12)	1.02	(0.92–1.13)
Balanced diet	1.01	(0.88–1.15)	1.04	(0.94–1.16)
Smoker	0.98	(0.56–1.72)	0.90	(0.59–1.36)
Health literacy	1.07	(0.79–1.43)	1.24†	(0.98–1.57)
Income	1.03	(0.95–1.12)	0.98	(0.82–1.05)
Health insurance	1.20	(0.61–2.34)	1.42	(0.84–2.40)
Urban	1.23	(0.78–1.94)	1.59*	(1.11–2.27)
Self-perceived health	0.88	(0.73–1.06)	0.97	(0.84–1.13)
Constant	0.01***	(0.00–0.12)	0.02***	(0.00–0.12)
Pseudo R^2	.103	(.095–.110)	.176	(.165–.186)
N		910		893

Source: National Public Opinion E-Health Survey, November 5-10, 2005.
*** p < .001; ** p < .01; * p < .05; †p < .10.

Table 6-2 reports results from logistic regression models predicting use of each type of website. We found that while older respondents were neither more nor less likely to visit government websites, they were less likely to visit private sector sites. In contrast, better educated respondents were more likely to seek information from both types of site.

Respondents with more negative attitudes toward health care access also were more likely to visit both public and private web locations. Whereas respondents with more negative attitudes toward health care affordability were more likely to visit private sector sites, they were neither more nor less likely to visit public sector ones.

There is evidence to suggest a relationship between stronger health literacy and urban or suburban residence and the probability of visiting a private sector website, but that was not the case with public sites. For the latter, neither place of residence nor health literacy affected the means of information acquisition.

We found no significant associations between usage of public or private sector websites and gender, race, insurance status, income, self-perceived health, lifestyle, and attitudes toward health care quality in general. There were few differences between men and women, whites and minorities, or poor and wealthy individuals. Each displayed the same visitation profile as its group counterpart.

CONCLUSION

The Internet is altering how people use health care services, obtain information, and evaluate alternatives. Where they acquire information, however, has implications for the quality of that information and the ability of technology to improve health care. Given the significant differences in various websites, it is crucial that policymakers understand where consumers go for health information.[4]

We found differences in the characteristics of public and private website users. On the one hand, our findings indicate that better educated respondents with more negative attitudes toward access were more likely to report visiting both public and private sponsor sites than less well educated respondents with more positive attitudes toward health care access.

On the other hand, the results indicate that younger respondents living in urban areas who had stronger health literacy and more negative attitudes toward affordability were more likely to visit privately sponsored sites. There was no relationship between age, health literacy, and attitudes toward affordability and use of government websites.

Analyses of previous website surveys found positive relationships between seeking health information over the Internet and being female, younger, or better educated; living in an urban or suburban location; and having a higher income.[5] Although not all of those relationships are reflected in the multivariate findings reported here (for example, those with respect to gender and income), all are reflected in the bivariate associations reported.[6]

Differences in website usage based on education, literacy, and residence illustrate the difficulties that policymakers face in closing the digital divide.[7] First, our results indicate that less well educated respondents exhibit a lower probability of accessing health information websites of any kind, implying the presence of a digital divide across both public and private sites. Second, they suggest that rural respondents with weaker health literacy are less likely to use private sector sites but neither more nor less likely to use public sector sites.

Although a digital divide exists, these patterns demonstrate that it is stronger and more pervasive in the private sector, where most information is written at a reading level well above that of many users. Many of the people who might benefit from going to commercial sites lack high-speed Internet or broadband access. The problem is especially relevant to e-health because needy beneficiaries are located predominantly in areas with limited Internet access, which makes its virtually impossible for them to take advantage of website content.[8]

The existence of different usage rates favoring private websites raises important questions regarding the type and quality of the information being downloaded. Eysenbach and colleagues and other researchers demonstrate that health information websites vary enormously in the validity of their information.[9] As we found in earlier chapters, some information presented on websites (especially commercial ones) is incomplete, inaccurate, or sponsored by interests with a financial stake in particular treatments. Private sector sites thus have the highest level of real or potential conflicts of interest owing to sponsorship by pharmaceutical or other health care companies.[10]

Website user characteristics provide further insights into other areas of digital medicine. Respondents with more negative attitudes toward health services were more likely to visit both government and private sector websites. That supports the expectation that individuals with greater difficulty accessing and/or affording care are more likely to seek alternative sources of online medical information, advice, and supplies. Younger respondents were more likely to get health information from private sector websites; however, they were neither more nor less likely to visit public sector sites. That implies that government websites may be posting less material directed toward younger age groups than private sector ones are.

At the time of the survey, the country's new Medicare Part D prescription drug benefit was nearing implementation.[11] The close proximity of that event and our survey may explain, in part, the findings reported here. Elderly individuals would have been especially motivated to visit websites, especially those of government agencies, because they needed to obtain information important to their future health care. Young people, in contrast, had no such motivation, and there was little that would have drawn them to government sites.

Our findings also relate to the idea that older people are less likely to use the Internet.[12] On average, older individuals have lower computer literacy than younger individuals. Indeed, seniors are much less likely than younger people to own a computer, let alone have access to the Internet.[13] Consequently, when seniors use the Internet, they may be more likely to do so at a senior center or public library, where the staff may be more inclined to steer them toward a public than a private sector website for certain services and information.

In contrast, younger people are more likely to access the Internet on their own, and they are more likely to rely on search engines such as Google. For individuals undertaking such searches, there is unlikely to be a predilection favoring some types of websites over others. However, since most websites are privately sponsored, it seems reasonable to conclude that younger respondents are guided to rely on a disproportionately larger number of private sites.

That younger people were more likely to visit private sector websites but not government websites is interesting also because they tend to be the most cynical about government in general. They are the bloc least likely to be engaged in the political process; for example, as an age group, young people vote about 30 percentage points less often than do senior citizens.[14]

That cynicism may extend to the Internet. If so, that is problematic, because private sector websites are more likely to show greater variability in content and to create more real or potential conflicts of interest. Younger individuals therefore may be at the greatest risk of receiving biased, one-sided, or incomplete health care information.

Since most commercial sites do not publicize the potential conflicts of interest created by outside ads or sponsorships, unwitting consumers may take the information presented at face value, not recognizing that it is sponsored by an interested party seeking to guide them toward particular choices. That danger is reflected in Internet searches of almost any disease or condition, which quickly reveal a plethora of sites that provide seemingly unbiased information but that are sponsored by pharmaceutical manufacturers presenting their own products in the best possible light.

Indeed, there are differences in the information screening processes used by government and nongovernment websites that affect website content.[15] A number of government agencies have advisory boards of experts who provide feedback on the agencies' decisions and the information that they provide. Although there is no guarantee that public sector information is always accurate, the fact that it goes through a screening process increases the odds that higher-quality and more accurate information will be provided online. The only cases in which that may not be the case occur in regard to highly politicized issues or when major differences of opinion exist among experts.

Furthermore, commercial sites are more likely to vary in the kind of material provided because their sponsors have incentives to promote products linked financially (or otherwise) to their organizational interests. They also differ in the types of marketing strategies employed. Government sites are marketed to the general public with little differentiation based on market segments. Although some material may be more relevant to some groups than others, as Medicare is to elderly or permanently disabled individuals, government officials do not target certain groups or emphasize niche marketing strategies.

In contrast, private sites sometimes follow niche strategies that allow them to focus their information resources on the desired audiences. They target particular groups on the basis of age, gender, race, income, interests, or other characteristics, attempting to match potential consumers with relevant products, information, or services.

Use of such a marketing strategy is found more often with for-profit than nonprofit websites. As Schlesinger and Gray observe in the context of health care in general, nonprofit and for-profit ownerships are distinct legal forms. Each has different operations, which "lead to different mixes of monetary and non-pecuniary incentives for administrators and staffs, different sources of capital, and different influences of governance."[16] In the world of digital medicine, variations in the end results of for-profit and nonprofit strategies are clearly seen. Different people tend to visit the different types of websites.

Unlike in many European countries, in which state-owned enterprises and corporatist governance structures remain common, in the United States there has long been a clear distinction between the public and private sectors that should enable people to distinguish between them at the electronic level. Since people can readily discern between the likes of Ford Motor Company and the U.S. Department of Transportation, Planned Parenthood and the Centers for Disease Control and Prevention, State Farm Insurance and the Federal Emergency Management Agency, and Merck Pharmaceuticals and the U.S. Food and Drug Administration, there is little reason to suspect that they would not know the difference between public and private sector websites as well.

People may readily differentiate between government and private websites, but they may find it harder to distinguish for-profit websites from not-for-profit sites. That difficulty should be kept in mind when comparing similarities and differences among Internet users visiting commercial and not-for-profit sites. Policymakers will not be able to close the digital divide until they understand the complex interplay among users' personal characteristics, website content, and website usage.

CHAPTER SEVEN

International Comparisons

A number of countries around the world have been successful at introducing technology into health care. The United Kingdom and New Zealand, for example, are far ahead of the United States in adoption of electronic health records by doctors: while 59 percent of the more than 30,000 health providers in the United Kingdom and 80 percent of the 9,000 doctors in New Zealand rely on electronic records, only 17 percent of the 650,000 physicians in the United States do so.[1]

Other nations have invested more than the United States in health information technology, putting considerable resources into developing high-speed broadband connections to link individuals and businesses to the Internet. For example, 35 percent of Danes but only 22 percent of Americans have access to high-speed broadband. That higher level of access has allowed site developers in such countries to put together high-quality websites that connect to one another and allow people from different areas to communicate. But the United States, which ranked fourth in broadband access among industrialized nations in 2001, dropped to fifteenth place in 2007.[2]

In locales such as Singapore and Malaysia, smart cards containing embedded circuits allow residents to complete a wide range of online transactions. These cards have holograms that prevent fraud, and the introduction of such cards has allowed agencies to place hundreds of official services online for use by citizens and businesses. Innovations in technology have extended even into the realm of transportation. Taxi drivers in Japan have advanced electronic systems that allow them to spot traffic delays, choose the most convenient routes, and find open parking spaces rather than circle the block, contributing to vehicular congestion.

A recent analysis of national government websites around the world found that the United States pales in comparison with countries such as South Korea and Taiwan in use of technology.[3] Along with high-speed broadband infrastructure, websites in the Asian countries offer a large number of electronic services, personalized content, media-rich applications, and easy access through PDA or handheld devices. Consequently, processing times are faster, download speeds are quicker, and Asian residents take less time to perform necessary functions.

This chapter presents studies of successful implementation of technology and also looks at the content of health department websites in various countries. We review cases in which foreign governments have incorporated technology into their health systems and analyze the content of government websites each year from 2001 to 2007. Our analyses cover the percentage of government websites that have privacy and security policies, the content of privacy policies, the percentage of health websites that can be accessed by disabled users, the number of health websites that provide access for speakers of foreign languages, and the percentage that run commercial advertising. We look at trends over time and compare Organization for Economic Cooperation and Development (OECD) countries with non-OECD nations to examine the impact of disparities in wealth on the development of health information technology.

Overall, we find that many non-U.S. public sector health sites lag behind those of U.S. state health departments on a variety of measures. The health sites of other locales, especially in non-OECD countries, are less likely to have privacy policies or provide various types of access. However, some countries in Asia and Europe have made innovative use of health information technology. The United Kingdom, Singapore, and Australia also present illuminating cases of technological innovation. In general, centralized government systems have had greater success in producing uniform standards and encouraging innovation in health technology than have decentralized systems such as those in the United States.

GLOBAL VARIATIONS IN INTERNET USAGE

Not all regions of the world share equally in the digital revolution. Table 7-1 demonstrates that Internet penetration levels are highest in North

TABLE 7-1. Internet Usage Levels by Region, 2007

Region	Population	Internet usage	Percent Internet usage of overall population
Africa	933,448,292	32,765,700	3.5
Asia	3,712,527,624	389,392,288	10.5
Europe	809,624,686	312,722,892	38.6
Middle East	193,452,727	19,382,400	10.0
North America	334,538,018	232,057,067	69.4
Latin America	556,606,627	88,778,986	16.0
Pacific Island area	34,468,443	18,430,359	53.5
Total	6,574,666,417	1,093,529,692	16.6

Source: Internet World Stats, 2007 (www.InternetWorldStats.com).

America (69.4 percent) and the Pacific Island areas (53.5 percent) and lowest in Africa (3.5 percent) and the Middle East (10 percent). Only 16.6 percent of the population of the world as a whole used the Internet in 2007, meaning that five-sixths of the planet's population is not participating in the digital revolution. Because many nations offer their people little access to health information technology, they are not able to gain the purported benefits of digital medicine; the absence of benefits, in turn, slows the diffusion of technology. The world's information divide therefore represents a major barrier to the successful use of technology in many health systems.

GLOBAL USE OF HEALTH INFORMATION TECHNOLOGY

As use of the Internet grows in various places around the world, there is increasing reliance on the World Wide Web for health care information. A recent general population poll of 7,934 people in Norway, Denmark, Germany, Greece, Poland, Portugal, and Latvia found that 44 percent of the total sample had employed the Internet for health purposes. Twenty-five percent indicated that they had employed the web to prepare for or to follow up after medical consultations. And when selecting health care providers, more than a third of the sample claimed that electronic provision of medical services was important to them. Those who most favored e-health services included young people, those with higher education, and white-collar employees.[4]

However, there is tremendous variation in use of health information technology across nations. A 2006 survey of primary care physicians by

TABLE 7-2. Health Care Performance Indicators in Seven Countries

Indicator	Australia	Great Britain	Canada	Germany	Nether-lands	New Zealand	United States
Health care spending as percent of GDP	9.5	8.3	9.8	10.7	9.2	9	16
Life expectancy (years)	80.6	78.7	80.3	79	79.8	79	77.9
Percent of patients believing medical system needs to be reformed	18	15	12	27	9	17	34
Percent of patients having experienced medical mistakes	26	24	28	16	25	22	32
Percent of patients getting appointment next day when sick	62	58	36	65	70	75	49

Source: Cathy Schoen and others, "Toward Higher-Performance Health Systems," *Health Affairs*, November 1, 2007.

the Harvard School of Public Health and the Commonwealth Fund found major differences across various countries in implementation of electronic medical records. For example, while just 17 percent of American doctors and 14 percent of Canadian medical professionals relied on electronic records, the numbers were higher in the United Kingdom (59 percent) and Australia (25 percent).

The study discovered furthermore that use of electronic prescribing by doctors ranged from 87 percent in the United Kingdom, 52 percent in New Zealand, and 44 percent in Australia to 9 percent in the United States and 8 percent in Canada.[5] Compared with some other nations, the United States obviously has a long way to go to reap the benefits of digital medicine.

However, there appears to be little correlation between the amount of money a country invests on health care and system performance indicators. As shown in table 7-2, the United States devotes the greatest percentage of gross domestic product (GDP) to health care (16 percent), but of the seven nations surveyed (Australia, Great Britain, Canada, Germany, Netherlands, New Zealand, and the United States), it has the lowest life expectancy.[6] The United States furthermore has the highest percentage of patients who believe that the medical system needs to be completely rebuilt; who have experienced medical mistakes in the past two years; and who have problems getting a doctor's appointment the next day when they become sick. That does not bode well for investment in health-related technology because ultimately people want to see a strong tie between public investment and health care outcomes.

As a sign of international interest in digital medicine, the World Health Organization (WHO) passed an e-health resolution in 2005 recognizing the importance of health information technology. The resolution represented an effort to coordinate member actions and provide a blueprint of related "norms, standards, guidelines, and information and training materials." The document not only sought to provide guidance on future development, it also addressed issues of equity and justice with respect to differences in wealth among nations and published a statement of e-health "rights and ethics." Among the principles promulgated in the resolution was that "efforts are needed to tackle the undue burden of ill-health borne by vulnerable and marginalized groups."[7] To monitor progress toward its goals, the WHO created a "global e-health observatory" charged with collecting data and informing policymakers about trends in this area.[8]

E-health in developing nations has become a particular challenge. As pointed out by Mohan and Suleiman, low-income nations have difficulty finding the resources necessary for investment in health technology. Few of their citizens use the Internet for any purpose, let alone health care; for example, 10 percent of people in Asia and the Middle East employ the Internet, while only 4 percent of those in Africa do so. Those areas cannot build information systems and justify the cost to citizens who lack basic services in education, health care, and transportation.[9]

To cope with such issues, the World Health Organization and the International Medical Informatics Association have formed an alliance to train health care workers and share e-health products. As stated by Geissbuhler, Haux, and Kwankam, it is important for nongovernmental organizations to join forces and focus their efforts at overcoming barriers to innovation in technology.[10] That would allow the organizations to create economies of scale and improve coordination among relevant organizations.

INNOVATION IN EUROPE

There is considerable interest in use of health information technology throughout Europe. A Eurobarometer survey found that Europeans and Americans are similar in relying more heavily on personal health care providers than on other sources for health information. When asked where they get the most medical information, 45 percent cited personal health care providers, followed by the Internet (23 percent), television (20 percent), and newspapers (7 percent).[11]

However, there is variation across the European Union. Reliance on the Internet for health information is highest in Denmark and the Netherlands (40 percent) and lowest in Greece, Spain, and Portugal (15 percent or less). A North/South split exists within the European Union in overall access to digital technology (similar to that seen in other aspects of civic life), and that split has ramifications for use of health technology. Southern European nations are poorer and have been slower than their Northern counterparts in joining the Internet revolution. Many of the wealthier Northern countries have invested substantially in digital communications; furthermore, they have better developed education systems, which correlates with improvements in information technology infrastructure and usage.

A number of European nations surpass the United States in reliance on information technology. In the United Kingdom, for example, more than 95 percent of family medical practices have computerized functions, ranging from extensive reliance on electronic medical records to use of computers for patient communication and referrals.[12] In 2004, the United Kingdom started a program called Connecting for Health that allows 50 million National Health Service (NHS) patients to have electronic health records. Under the program, all of an individual's medical information is summarized in a single database and the NHS's 30,000 physicians are given access to that material.[13]

Currently, there are four major e-health initiatives under way in the United Kingdom. Doctors are using a videoconferencing system to connect different medical facilities; hospitals are providing bedside laptop systems for patient-doctor communications; outpatients are relying on digital devices to monitor specific diseases; and physicians are using electronic monitoring devices to aid patients with certain ailments.[14]

Despite significant progress, privacy remains a major concern for the public at large. A survey by the British Medical Association found that 75 percent of respondents indicated that they would not mind having a central computer hold their medical information but that 75 percent also worried about information security in a national database. As do consumers in the United States, British consumers fear that their confidential records will be compromised, and policymakers are devising security measures and audit trails to reduce the risk of unauthorized access to medical records.

Other European nations also have placed a priority on health information technology. Use of electronic technology in Germany has been rising. In 2001, a survey of young people ages 15 to 28 revealed that 27 percent used the Internet to gather health information. However, by 2005, the number had virtually doubled, to 53 percent, among the same age group.[15]

But other e-health avenues have been slow to develop in Germany. Only 6 percent of Germans said that they had e-mailed their health care professional, 2 percent indicated that they had used e-mail or the Internet to renew a prescription, and 2 percent said that they had used the Internet to schedule a medical appointment. That demonstrates that slow adoption of digital medicine is not limited to the United States, where the figures for those functions were similar.

One of the reasons for limited progress in some European countries has been low investment in information technology. A Health Information Network study of hospitals in fifteen European nations found that they spend only 1.8 percent of their overall budget on information technology, a figure similar to that for comparable hospitals in the United States. Failure to devote greater financial resources makes it difficult for some European nations to take full advantage of technology's benefits.[16]

This problem also shows up in figures for medical ordering systems. Overall, only 2.2 percent of European medical facilities have adopted computerized physician order entry systems; the U.S. figure is 2.5 percent.[17] Until financial investments increase, European countries will not be able to bring the digital revolution home to their residents.

But usage is expected to increase. In 2006, about 1 percent of total health care budgets in the European Union went toward electronic health features. By 2010, however, that figure is projected to rise to 5 percent among the twenty-five member nations. Overall, 78 percent of general practitioners in the European Union are online, with the highest use occurring in Sweden (98 percent) and the United Kingdom (97 percent).[18] That demonstrates that the potential for an e-health revolution is quite high, at least in some European countries.

INNOVATION IN CANADA

Canada is moving forward with ambitious plans to computerize its health care facilities. The provinces of Alberta and New Brunswick have signed contracts with a private company, CGI Group, to develop a "one person, one record" electronic database.[19] New Brunswick has agreed to spend about C$250 million over the next ten years to connect patients and specialists through electronic devices.[20] The region's goal is to deploy online learning programs to inform people about how to access medical care and survive health pandemics.

New technology has been used to enfranchise marginalized populations. One of the chief virtues of electronic communications is its ability to overcome social and geographical distances. For example, Canada provides satellite broadcasting and telemedicine for the Inuit, an indigenous group that is scattered across wide, rural regions. The Inuit have long complained that they were excluded from new technologies and subjected to "colonizing" influences from the central government. Now, the Internet, satellite communications, and telemedicine are available to the Inuit, who are able to communicate with health professionals in their native language and get medical advice tailored to their particular group.[21]

Hospitals in Ontario have installed bedside terminals manufactured by the Telus Corporation that provide Internet access to patients and doctors and allow them to access electronic medical records. The terminals also make television available on demand and allow patients to order room service.[22]

Overall, the Canadian government has spent more than C$1.2 billion on health technology. Public officials at Health Canada Infoway, the agency in charge of e-health services, have high hopes for that investment. Government authorities claim that further use of health information technology will save Canadians C$6 billion a year.[23]

The fact that Canada is investing substantial resources in electronic health services bodes well for its long-run prospects. Once high-speed communication lines are put in place, it will be easier for hospitals and doctors to built health-related content, and private companies can develop software systems knowing that there is sufficient broadband capacity to support the systems.

The centralized nature of the Canadian health care system has speeded technological progress, particularly through the adoption of uniform national standards. Health care providers in different regions rely on similar systems. Commercial developers know that they must develop health information systems that are interoperable and connect easily to systems made by other vendors; if their systems do not communicate well with other hardware, the national health system will not authorize purchase of the equipment.

Neither Canada nor the United Kingdom faces a fragmented health care system like that in the United States. Centralization produces more coherent health information technology than decentralization. However, unitary systems do not solve all the problems with technological innovation. Budget constraints and reservations on the part of consumers remain, along with challenges in overcoming providers' resistance and the digital divide. But having an institutional setting that reduces fragmentation appears to speed innovation.

INNOVATION IN ASIA

Singapore, Hong Kong, and Taiwan are the e-health leaders in Asia. Singapore has technology that allows patients to make medical appointments online, access their medical records, order drugs online, and share information with medical professionals.[24] The health care section within that nation's eCitizen website provides general health care information, maintains a list of health care providers, and allows for a wide variety of online medical transactions.

Taiwan operates an e-hospital website through the Ministry of Health that provides free online advice to patients regarding a variety of illnesses. Patients submit their questions through the website and receive answers either through the site or by e-mail from medical practitioners and nutritionists at the country's various hospitals.

Hong Kong's national health authority has introduced an innovative online networking system for hospitals that allows patients and doctors to communicate online, provides electronic medical records for doctors and patients, and speeds communication among health care providers.

Meanwhile, Japan is falling behind its Asian counterparts in online health services. It does not provide the range of digital medical services available in other countries, nor has it invested as much as South Korea, Taiwan, and Singapore in broadband infrastructure. The result has been slow computer communications and a private sector that has not invested major sums of money in health information technology.

In 2007, however, Nagoya University Hospital launched a new Fujitsu Primequest server that speeds access to patient records and integrates them with the hospital's accounting, examination, radiology, and surgical systems. This hospital was the first in Japan to launch an online medical records system a few years ago and has long been a leader in technological innovation.[25] Japanese leaders hope that the new electronic system will speed use of technology and give patients and doctors readier access to up-to-date medical information.

In China, an alliance between IBA Health and Shanghai People's Health Information Technology Company will create a national health-related television channel on the country's Internet protocol television network. The channel will allow doctors and patients to conduct medical consultations over the Internet from different geographical locations. The Shanghai company also has installed information technology systems in 180 hospitals around Shanghai as a way to boost the productivity of its health care system.[26]

Despite some noteworthy exceptions, China lags behind other Asian nations in technological innovation. For example, only about 10 percent of its people have access to the Internet. But the country is investing more of its growing wealth in broadband development and electronic systems, offering increasing hope that China will be able to bring digital medicine to more of its citizens in the near future.

People in Southeast Asia have long suffered from an HIV/AIDS epidemic fueled by a large sex industry. But now, digital technologies are being used to bring preventive medicine to those in need. The UN program on HIV/AIDS has created an information development project with the World Bank that publicizes digital medicine resources in developing countries in an effort to link patients and health care providers through e-mail and other digital devices.[27]

INNOVATION IN AUSTRALIA

In Australia, the national E-Health Transition Authority, funded by the Council of Australian Governments, is devoting A$130 billion to the development of an electronic health record system; it also has developed national standards to guide development of the records.[28] In addition, the national Council on Health and Aging maintains eGuild, an online pharmacy that serves patients across the country.[29] Government contractors now have to demonstrate that their information systems can connect to those of other vendors before they win a contract; in the past, public authorities took the word of private suppliers that their systems were interoperable.[30]

Australia also is home to IBA Health Limited, which is one of the world's largest health information technology providers. IBA operates more than 13,000 health care systems in the United Kingdom, Ireland, continental Europe, Africa, the Middle East, Asia, Australia, and New Zealand, handling administrative systems as well as electronic records.[31]

All of this technological innovation appears to have influenced consumer behavior. A survey in Australia found that 83 percent of patients said that information that they found on the Internet had influenced the questions that they asked their doctors. Twenty-one percent indicated that they had found information online that their doctor was not aware of, and 18 percent said that online information had led them to alter a health care decision.[32]

However, many of those surveyed did not trust information found on the Internet. When asked whether they trusted their doctor more than the Internet, 88 percent said yes. Only 5 percent said that they trusted the Internet more, and 7 percent were unsure. Twenty-three percent said that they always believed that information found on the Internet was correct, and 77 percent said that they sometimes believed that the material was correct.[33]

One emerging problem in the era of new technology concerns identity fraud. A national survey found that 10 percent of Australians claimed that they had been the victim of identity theft in the previous year. Forty-five percent believed that identity theft was likely to take place when people used the Internet, and half of those interviewed indicated that they were more worried about giving confidential information over the Internet than they were two years before. Indeed, such concerns are serious enough that Australia now sponsors Privacy Awareness Week during August of each year to promote sensitivity to privacy risks. The initiative is evidence of the powerful role that citizens' concerns about security and privacy play in electronic health.[34] Unless national governments take those concerns seriously, they will compromise the future of digital medicine, which will lead to slower development than would otherwise occur.

INNOVATION IN AFRICA

Africa is the region least likely to participate in the information technology revolution. Given widespread poverty, the weakness of the health system, and the inefficiency of the public sector, it has been difficult to develop viable electronic resources. Barriers to use of technology predominate across all forty-five countries of Africa. For example, for the continent as a whole, the adult literacy rate averages 61 percent, and only 29 percent of the population has been enrolled in secondary school. In addition, only 3 percent of the people have telephone landlines; only 6 percent have cell phones; and only 1.6 percent report using the Internet. Moreover, average annual income per capita is just $3,158.[35]

The overall weakness of Africa's economic and communications infrastructure makes it nearly impossible to develop telemedicine or electronic health services. There simply is little way for patients to consult with doctors other than through in-person visits. E-mailing health care providers is not viable, only the most elite individuals can access health care information over the Internet, and electronic medical records do not exist.

The nonexistence of an electronic communications system makes it difficult to be optimistic about the future of digital medicine in Africa. According to research undertaken by several scholars, there is a strong association between income, education, and use of telecommunications.[36] Countries whose residents have low education and income generally do not have telephones, personal computers, or Internet access. Therefore, if nations wish to boost use of telecommunications, they need economic development strategies that increase education and income levels. If they do that, it will become easier for Africans to make use of digital medicine.

ONLINE SERVICES AT NATIONAL HEALTH DEPARTMENT WEBSITES

These cross-national examples demonstrate that there is wide variation around the world in access to health information technology but that people in many nations have common fears about online privacy and security regarding medical records. Poverty and inequality clearly have limited the progress of some nations; furthermore, a variety of political, institutional, and cultural forces have slowed e-health progress in many places, just as in the United States.

In order to conduct a more systematic comparison of national health department websites, we undertook a detailed content analysis of such sites in a cross-section of sixty-six nations around the world (see appendix C for the list of websites). Countries from developed and developing nations were included, as were the different regions of the world. When the website was not in English, we relied on translations.

TABLE 7-3. Percent of National Health Department Websites with Online Services, OECD and Non-OECD Countries

Countries	2001	2002	2003	2004	2005	2006	2007
Overall ($N = 66$)	4	11	15	25	22	29	25
OECD countries ($N = 30$)	0	21	24	40	27	41	40
Non-OECD countries ($N = 36$)	4	6	11	19	20	24	17

Source: Authors' e-health content analysis, 2001–07.

Among the items that we explored were interactive features, online reports and databases, reading level, access for speakers of foreign languages, access for disabled users, commercial advertising, and the presence of privacy and security statements. We focused on those features because of their importance for access to and the reliability of technology.

We compared online features to see how countries rate in the use of digital technology on their health websites and analyzed websites from 2001 to 2007 to see what longitudinal trends were present. Comparing sites over time helped us determine which countries were innovating and which had made the most rapid progress.

Table 7-3 shows a general trend toward an increase in websites offering online services. In 2001, when we first examined health websites, only 4 percent provided any services on their sites; the number grew to 29 percent in 2006, although it dropped to 25 percent in 2007. Among the features found on government websites were reports on hospital quality, online health benefits forms, and searchable databases of physicians with particular specialties.

To measure the impact of wealth and overall development on the availability of electronic health services, we compared thirty Organization for Economic Cooperation and Development (OECD) nations and thirty-six non-OECD countries. The OECD nations included Australia, Austria, Belgium, Canada, the Czech Republic, Denmark, Finland, France, Germany, Greece, Hungary, Iceland, Ireland, Italy, Japan, Korea, Luxembourg, Mexico, Netherlands, New Zealand, Norway, Poland, Portugal, Slovakia, Spain, Sweden, Switzerland, Turkey, the United Kingdom, and the United States.

As one would expect, the OECD nations were much more likely than their non-OECD counterparts to offer online services. In 2007, for example, 40 percent of health sites in OECD countries but only 17 percent in non-OECD nations had online services. In general, wealthier

TABLE 7-4. Percent of National Health Department Websites Having Privacy and Security Policies, OECD and Non-OECD Countries

Policy	2001	2002	2003	2004	2005	2006	2007
Privacy policy							
Overall	7	13	15	14	21	31	32
OECD countries	20	16	36	28	32	54	52
Non-OECD countries	5	11	6	8	16	20	21
Security policy							
Overall	4	11	10	5	8	18	22
OECD countries	10	16	24	4	9	29	40
Non-OECD countries	3	9	4	6	7	12	13

Source: Authors' e-health content analysis, 2001–07.

nations were at least twice as likely to have health departments providing online services as countries with more limited financial resources.

PRIVACY AND SECURITY

There is a growing trend toward posting privacy and security policies online. Citizens in many countries worry about the confidentiality and security of health websites, and a number of well-publicized security breaches have reinforced public concerns, leading governments to take those concerns much more seriously. As countries modernize, the threat of unauthorized disclosure of confidential information becomes more worrisome to many people.

As shown in table 7-4, only 7 percent of national government health websites had a privacy policy in 2001; however, the number rose to 32 percent in 2007. Similarly, the number of sites having a security policy rose from 4 percent in 2001 to 22 percent in 2007, demonstrating that government health sites are making progress on these key performance indicators.

OECD nations were much more likely than non-OECD nations to have website privacy and security policies. In 2007, 52 percent of OECD nations but only 21 percent of non-OECD nations had a privacy policy. A similar pattern was seen for security policies: 40 percent of OECD countries but only 13 percent of non-OECD nations had a security policy in 2007.

TABLE 7-5. Percent of National Health Department Websites Having Privacy Policies

Policy	2002	2003	2004	2005	2006	2007
Prohibits commercial marketing	9	12	10	12	23	25
Prohibits cookies	6	4	4	9	4	12
Prohibits sharing of personal information	11	12	10	9	21	25
Permits sharing of personal information with law enforcement agencies	7	8	9	6	23	13

Source: Authors' e-health content analysis, 2002–07.

We also examined the quality of national health department privacy policies. While improvements were made from 2001 to 2007, most countries do not safeguard consumer privacy interests very comprehensively. For example, in 2007, only 25 percent of online health site privacy policies prohibited the commercial marketing of visitor information, 12 percent prohibited cookies, 25 percent prohibited sharing personal information, and 13 percent said that they shared information with law enforcement officials (see table 7-5). Those results suggest that there is much more work to be done in the area of safeguarding confidential medical records.

ACCESS FOR DISABLED INDIVIDUALS

As in the United States, progress has been slow in other nations on providing access to health website information for disabled individuals. For example, in 2005, only 25 percent of health sites could be accessed by the disabled, up from 18 percent in 2003. OECD countries (52 percent) were more likely than non-OECD nations (11 percent) to have accessible sites (see table 7-6). But overall, much greater progress needs to be made to help the disabled access government health care information.

TRANSLATION INTO FOREIGN LANGUAGES

Another measure of website accessibility is language. Many countries have citizens who do not speak the native language, and it is helpful to provide information for them in their own language (see table 7-7). In 2007, 60 percent of health department sites provided translation into foreign languages. OECD countries (72 percent) were more likely than

TABLE 7-6. Percent of National Health Department Websites Providing Access for Disabled Users, OECD and Non-OECD Countries

Percent

Countries	2003	2004	2005	2006	2007
Overall	18	14	18	20	25
OECD countries	36	32	36	50	52
Non-OECD countries	9	6	9	6	11

Source: Authors' e-health content analysis, 2003–07.

non-OECD countries (53 percent) to do so, again demonstrating the importance of differences in wealth in addressing access issues.

COMMERCIAL ADVERTISING

Commercial advertising is rarely found on health department websites. For example, only 1 percent of such sites (none of the OECD country sites and only 2 percent of non-OECD country sites) ran commercial ads in 2007. Because most national government health websites are financed by general taxes, advertisements are not commonly used to raise revenue for the sites.

Excluding ads is a desirable practice because it helps consumers avoid real or potential conflicts of interest. Users are not being bombarded with advertisements at most public sector sites, so they do not have to worry about compromised information or biased presentations (see table 7-8). Of course, in developing nations, many consumers go not to public sector sites but to private ones, which are far more likely to have sponsored links or product commercials.

OVERALL COUNTRY RANKINGS

To compare how countries are using technology overall on their national health department websites, we analyzed the sites of sixty-six nations around the world. We created a 100-point e-government index and ranked each nation's health department website on the basis of the availability of publications and databases and the number of online services offered. Four points were awarded to each website for each of the following features: publications, databases, audio clips, video clips, foreign language access, no ads, no premium fees, no user fees, access

TABLE 7-7. Percent of National Health Department Websites Providing Translation into Foreign Languages, OECD and Non-OECD Countries
Percent

Countries	2001	2002	2003	2004	2005	2006	2007
Overall	39	32	46	42	40	45	60
OECD countries	70	52	64	72	54	67	72
Non-OECD countries	35	20	38	28	33	34	53

Source: Authors' e-health content analysis, 2001–07.

for disabled users, privacy policies, security policies, acceptance of digital signatures on transactions, a credit card payment option, e-mail contact information, an area for posting comments, an option for e-mail updates, options for website personalization, and PDA access. A maximum of seventy-two points could be awarded to each website for including those features.

Each site could then qualify for another twenty-eight points, depending on the number of online services the site offered (one point for one service, two points for two services, three points for three services, and up to twenty-eight points for twenty-eight or more services). Adding these elements together, the e-government index ran from zero points (having none of the features and no online services) to 100 (having all features plus at least twenty online services).

On the basis of this analysis, the top national health department websites in 2007 belonged to South Korea, Taiwan, the United States, Turkey, Canada, Great Britain, Malta, Spain, Ireland, and Brazil. The nations whose sites performed most poorly were Tanzania, Kuwait, Chile, Algeria, Thailand, and Paraguay. Table 7-9 lists the rankings of the sixty-six countries, which show that OECD nations generally performed better on e-health provision. Their health sites averaged 37.4 points and the non-OECD nations averaged 30.3 points overall on the 100-point scale. However, it is clear from the poor performance of both sets of countries that many nations need to make greater progress on technological innovation in the health care area.

PREDICTORS OF E-HEALTH PERFORMANCE

We have described e-health performance in various countries around the world, but we have not explained the variation that exists. Clearly, some

TABLE 7-8. Percent of National Health Department Websites Having Advertisements, OECD and Non-OECD Countries

Percent

Countries	2001	2002	2003	2004	2005	2006	2007
Overall	1	9	0	0	3	0	1
OECD countries	0	0	0	0	0	0	0
Non-OECD countries	1	14	0	0	4	0	2

Source: Authors' e-health content analysis, 2001–07.

nations have done better at implementing health information technology than others, and it is important to understand why those places have performed more effectively than others.

We have argued that a variety of technological, social, political, and economic forces are important for innovation in digital technology. In our content analysis as well as our investigation of public opinion, we have suggested that party affiliation, social background, financial costs, and access to technology affect whether people use digital health services. Those factors influence how individuals see new technologies as well as their willingness to make use of electronic options.

In order to determine the reasons behind global e-health performance, we regressed our score of national government health department websites on technological, social, political, and fiscal factors. Technological features included international Internet bandwidth measured as bits per person, number of broadband subscribers per 1,000 people, and number of Internet users per 1,000 people. Societal health was measured by the percentage of a country's population immunized for diphtheria at ages 12 to 23 months, percent immunized for measles at ages 12 to 23 months, number malnourished (in millions), and mortality rate for children under the age of 5 per 1,000 people.[37]

Health capacity was measured through health expenditures per capita, health expenditures as a percentage of gross domestic product, hospital beds per 1,000 people, and physicians per 1,000 people. Political factors were measured through the Freedom House civil liberties score and the Tatu Vanhanen measure of political competition (percentage of legislative seats controlled by the major party). Economic factors were measured through each nation's per capita GDP in current U.S. dollars.[38]

Table 7-10 shows the results of this analysis. Overall, our model explained about one-quarter of the variation in e-health performance. The most significant factors in determining a country's website content

TABLE 7-9.   Ranking of National Government Health Department Websites, 2007

Country	Score	Country	Score	Country	Score
South Korea	79	Lebanon	34	India	28
Taiwan	64	Malaysia	32	Iraq	28
United States	59	Norway	32	Israel	28
Turkey	52	Saudi Arabia	32	Jamaica	28
Canada	51	Belgium	32	Kenya	28
Great Britain	49.5	China	32	Luxembourg	24
Malta	49	France	32	Mauritius	24
Spain	49	Iceland	32	Nicaragua	24
Ireland	48	Japan	32	Philippines	24
Brazil	47	Mexico	30	Poland	24
Switzerland	45	Sweden	29	Senegal	24
New Zealand	44	Lesotho	28	South Africa	24
Bahrain	44	Qatar	28	Zimbabwe	24
Peru	44	Slovenia	28	El Salvador	24
Singapore	44	Syria	28	Argentina	24
Australia	41.7	Ukraine	28	Hungary	24
Denmark	40	Vietnam	28	Paraguay	20
Germany	37	Cuba	28	Thailand	20
Maldives	36	Estonia	28	Algeria	20
Hong Kong	36	Fiji	28	Chile	20
Iran	36	Finland	28	Kuwait	20
Panama	35	Arab Emirates	28	Tanzania	16

Source: Tabulations based on authors' e-health content analysis, 2007.

were the number of broadband users and the mortality rate for children under the age of 5 years. The more broadband users, the more likely the country was to have a strong health department website; the worse the mortality rate, the more likely it was to have a weak site.

No political or economic forces were statistically significant. It did not matter how liberal the nation was with respect to civil liberties or how much political competition existed. Nor did it matter how wealthy the country was or how strong its health care infrastructure was, as measured by health expenditures. Those factors bore no significant relationship to e-health performance at the national level.

CONCLUSION

To summarize, we found wide variation in use of health information technology across national boundaries. Non-OECD nations lag behind OECD nations on a variety of technology measures. For example, they

TABLE 7-10. Logistic Regression of Technology and Social, Political, and Economic Forces on E-Health Performance, 2007

International bandwith capacity	.00	(.00)
Number of broadband subscribers	.11	(.04)**
Number of Internet users	.01	(.01)
Health expenditures per capita	−.00	(.00)
Health expenditures as a percent of GDP	1.46	(.96)
Number of hospital beds	−.85	(.72)
Percent of population immunized against diptheria	−.05	(.34)
Percent of population immunized against measles	−.10	(.28)
Number of malnourished people	.00	(.06)
Mortality rate	−.11	(.06)*
Number of physicians	−1.99	(1.80)
Civil liberties index	.32	(1.22)
Political competition	−.06	(.10)
GDP per capita	−00	(.00)
Constant	42.2	(24.5)*
Adjusted R^2	22 percent	
F score	2.265**	
N	65	

Source: Tabulations based on authors' e-health content analysis, 2007.
$**p < .01; *p < .10.$

are less likely to have privacy policies, offer online services, or provide various types of access. However, within the OECD countries, places such as the United Kingdom, Singapore, and Australia have made significant progress, and in some cases their medical professionals have outpaced those in the United States. E-health performance is most affected by the number of broadband subscribers in a nation and its child mortality rate.

Generally, where health information technology has been widely used, a centralized regime, authoritarian political system, or unitary government has made technological innovation a national priority. A strong political will appears to be necessary to surmount bureaucratic resistance, marshal financial resources, and overcome partisan differences in a way that makes it possible for innovation to take place.

In such nations, the political and economic divisions that have slowed progress in the United States have been overcome and coalitions assembled to move toward greater use of information technology. That suggests that to make progress on digital medicine, public officials need to marshal the political will necessary and build coalitions to overcome organizational tendencies that impede technological innovation. Decentralized political systems face even greater challenges in introducing new technologies than more centralized institutional structures.

In order to move forward, governments need to invest money in broadband infrastructure and develop consistent national standards that allow health care providers and commercial vendors to produce systems that can link to others. In the world of health care today, interoperability is the word. With a wide range of health care clinicians and providers, it is important that investments in technology rest on comparable standards and communication technologies. Systems that connect well with one another make it easier for consumers to draw on the wealth of medical expertise that exists around the world.

CHAPTER EIGHT

Improving Digital Medicine

Our research has shown that public use of health information technology remains low; that there is little positive association between technology use and consumer attitudes about the health care system; that commercial websites typically have more ads, weaker disclosure, and greater conflicts of interest than government sites; and that a large segment of the general population (both in the United States and around the world) is not participating in the digital revolution. Together, those results cast doubt on the ability of health officials to achieve, in the short run, the service improvements, cost savings, and productivity gains desired through electronic health resources.

In this chapter, we focus on ways to improve digital medicine and reduce the disparities in the employment of health information technology. We examine a number of different approaches, such as improving education, boosting individuals' computer literacy, providing low-cost laptops or personal digital assistants to broaden access, investing in broadband infrastructure, training medical professionals in the use of new technologies, overcoming legal and political obstacles to wider usage, and taking ethics and the right to privacy seriously.

Basically, we argue that technology in itself will not improve medical care unless consumers and health care providers obtain training and infrastructure assistance to lower the barriers to broader usage. Efforts to encourage use of electronic health services must include infrastructure development, financial incentives to promote innovation, and education and training.[1] Although programs directed at facilitating usage need to target health care consumers, they also must work with medical providers. Unless prevailing obstacles with respect to communications, costs, confidentiality, and digital disparities are addressed, the depth and breadth of the e-health revolution will remain limited.[2]

We are optimistic about the future of digital medicine.[3] It still is early in the technology revolution, but our research suggests that with constructive policy adjustments and improved training, use of health information technology will increase and thereby help to transform service delivery and citizen attitudes about health care, even among those who might otherwise be least likely to use it. The key for policymakers is to adopt strategies to educate consumers, train medical providers, and close the digital divide in order to reap maximum benefits.

IMPROVING EDUCATION

Many people are not engaged in digital technologies. In the United States, nearly one-third of the population does not have access to computers and another third uses new technology irregularly. A 2006 Pew Internet and American Life Project classified Americans into elite tech users (31 percent), middle-of-the-road tech users (20 percent), and those having few tech assets (49 percent). In breaking the numbers down, Pew researchers found that only 8 percent of the population are "information omnivores," or active participants in the information society. Fifteen percent are completely off the network, 11 percent are indifferent to information technology, 15 percent are light users, and 8 percent are inexperienced with digital technology.[4]

Around the world, a startling 83 percent of the total population does not have access to or use the Internet for any purpose.[5] For people who are poor, uneducated, or elderly or who live in rural areas, it is as if computers were never invented. Such individuals do not surf the web and do not worry about the inconvenience of a temporary loss of their wireless connection. They have no access to electronic health resources or any other online services.

As long as large segments of the population remain detached from the digital revolution, it will prove impossible to achieve widespread use of electronic medical records, use of e-mail for doctor-patient communications, or development of sophisticated websites that include detailed health care information. Those outside the digital world will not take advantage of new technologies and will not gain the benefits of digital medical services.[6] They will continue to engage predominantly in face-to-face contact with medical providers, and it will be virtually impossible to reform the health care system in a comprehensive manner through digital technology.

Since greater use of technology is highly correlated with greater education, boosting literacy and knowledge represents one key to improving access to technology and use of digital medical resources. From the standpoint of technological literacy, education has many virtues. One multi-country study found that the perceived usefulness of computers rose as individuals' level of literacy increased. As people became more informed, they were able to understand why computers were helpful and were able to learn how to use digital resources to perform specific tasks. That was true even after age and income were taken into account.[7]

Literacy is especially important in medical care because it is connected with a wide variety of disease and treatment outcomes. Medical researchers have found that individuals with limited literacy have less detailed information about diseases, are less likely to employ common kinds of preventive health measures, and experience poorer health overall.[8] For such individuals, literacy is not an abstract concept but one that correlates with highly desirable health outcomes.[9]

As pointed out earlier, not everyone has the same opportunity to use health information technology. Among the groups least likely to rely on digital medical resources are people who are elderly, low income, or poorly educated or who live in rural areas. Individuals with low income and poor education simply do not have access to the technology revolution and thus have been unable to benefit from recent advances in electronic medicine. Economics is a big part of the problem. According to national statistics, while 37 percent of families making more than $30,000 have ready access to the Internet, among those making less than $30,000, only 18 percent have access.[10]

At the other end of the spectrum are Asian Americans, who are the group most likely to have access to the Internet and to make use of digital resources. It is estimated that 75 percent of this group have access to the Internet, a percentage that is far higher than that found with other socioeconomic groups.[11] This set of individuals has considerable economic resources and sees great virtue in Internet communications technology.

Interestingly, there is a significant gender gap in favor of females. Women are more likely than men to surf the web for medical information and to make health care decisions for their families.[12] Among the activities of great interest to women are searching for health information online and using e-mail to communicate with health care providers.[13] They see extensive benefits to electronic health and are more likely than men to take advantage of online medical information.

BOOSTING COMPUTER LITERACY

Once people gain access to computers and the Internet, it is important to boost their skillfulness in taking advantage of digital resources. Not all people feel equally comfortable searching for information online. Many worry that they will lose valuable benefits from medical providers if they rely on virtual contact instead of face-to-face visits.[14] A survey found that 42 percent of the general population in the United States is not happy with having to respond to electronic devices, such as computers, cell phones, and e-mail.[15]

More specifically, consumers cite a number of barriers that make them reluctant to use electronic health resources. According to researchers, 39 percent of people worry about the privacy of the Internet, 29 percent say that they have difficulty evaluating the accuracy of online materials, 26 percent report that their physician disapproves of use of online health resources, 18 percent say that online information is inaccurate, and 13 percent find Internet content unreliable.[16]

Clearly, if consumers feel that information obtained online is inaccurate, they are not likely to trust or make use of online materials. Confidence in both the technology and online content is required if people are to see electronic resources as a valuable complement to or substitute for face-to-face encounters. If they consider online material questionable, they are not going to look for it in the future.

Young people in particular are especially sensitive to privacy concerns. Many of them go online for confidential health care information. They may be interested in finding out about sexually transmitted diseases or drug or alcohol issues. According to focus groups, those who worry that their search is not confidential become less likely to rely on the Internet for health information.[17]

It is crucial, therefore, to offer training on how to search for information online and ways to evaluate its overall quality. One study of King County, Washington, residents found that unfamiliarity with digital technology was rated equally as important as cost as a barrier to digital usage among women. For example, 38 percent cited computer affordability as a reason for not accessing health care information on the Internet, 36 percent indicated that they did not know how to use the Internet, 34 percent said that they could not pay the monthly access fee, and 33 percent felt that the Internet was not useful.[18] If people find technology intimidating or are not sure how to search Internet sites, they are less likely to take advantage of digital health resources.

PROVIDING LOW-COST TECHNOLOGY

Recognizing that not everyone has equal access to digital technology, some nonprofit organizations have worked to facilitate access. For example, there have been efforts to develop low-cost laptops for poor people. A nonprofit organization called One Laptop Per Child offers new computers (XO laptops) for $350, designed for people living in impoverished countries.

The computers use free Linux open-source software, and they have wireless capability and a built-in camera; in addition, they are manufactured to withstand the severe weather conditions common in parts of Africa, Asia, and Latin America. The devices are waterproof and have screens that can be viewed in direct sunlight. They operate on a hand-cranked battery that can last for up to twelve hours.[19]

Early reviews of the XO laptops have been very positive. Engineers describe them as "light, rugged and surprisingly versatile." Focus group testing has revealed that children like to use them and find them easy to navigate. One young tester gave the machine the ultimate compliment by describing it as "completely beastly."[20]

However, orders have lagged expectations. The organization's leaders thought that there would be requests for 3 million machines, but the actual number has been far lower. Governments in Peru, Mexico, and Uruguay have ordered laptops for distribution in rural areas. Italy has purchased devices for distribution in Ethiopia. But expected large orders from Nigeria and Brazil failed to come through. The price of the machines continued to exceed what people in developing nations were willing to pay. Foundation officials responded by launching a two-for-one promotion in which donors could buy one for a poor child in a developing nation and get another free for their personal use.[21] However, orders still have not come in at the anticipated rate.

Other countries have sought to bypass desktop computing by moving digital access directly to cell phones or personal digital assistant (PDA) devices. The virtue of such units is their low cost, mobility, and ease of use for people who are not well versed in computing technology. Even in poor nations, cell phones have become widely used. The World Bank estimates that 18 percent of the population in low- and middle-income countries have a mobile phone, whereas just 4 percent have a personal computer.[22] If impoverished countries want to get digital medical resources to their citizens, it makes sense for them to employ the mobile technologies currently in use in their area.

Wireless technology offers the virtue of relatively low cost; it takes an investment of only a few hundred dollars to purchase a cell phone or wireless device. By providing electronic access at an affordable price, this kind of technology lowers the economic barrier to broader use and makes it possible for more people to gain digital access.[23]

In health care, personal digital assistants are helpful not just for consumers but for health care providers, enabling doctors to file prescription orders and check online directories for proper medications and interaction effects while making patient rounds. Using this technology, medical personnel can communicate with patients, schedule appointments, or arrange for electronic consultations. Little training is required, and most health care professionals already are comfortable using these kinds of devices.

One study of PDA users among medical professionals found that the devices were an effective clinical tool. A small sample of doctors was given Palm PDAs along with software presenting various kinds of medical information. About half reported that they had been able to respond to specific questions because of the ability to run a digital search of a medical database. Overall, 92 percent reported that they found the Palm devices to provide useful support of their activities.[24]

The United Nations Internet Communications Technology taskforce has undertaken a global initiative to promote wireless networks in urban areas around the world.[25] UN officials hope that wireless connections, considered a "leapfrog" technology, will allow underserved populations to gain access to the Internet and thereby reap the advantages of information technology. If successful, the project will help those currently lacking access to the Internet to get connected.

INVESTING IN BROADBAND INFRASTRUCTURE

Broadband access is crucial to the future of electronic medicine. Health care providers cannot read X-rays or transfer electronic medical records without high-speed communication networks. Patients cannot watch the information videos now becoming more common at health care websites without broadband access. Slow-speed connections are not fast enough to support the needs of a modern health care system. They frustrate health care providers and forestall the efficiency gains desired by health policy reformers.

In countries where there has been a substantial leap forward on e-health, broadband investment has been a major factor. In the nineteenth and twentieth centuries, governments invested large sums of money in railroads, canals, highways, and airports. Those infrastructure investments spurred economic development, facilitated international commerce, and allowed business people to travel easily and communicate with customers and other business people.[26]

Governments in Asia and in some European countries have taken responsibility for building technology infrastructure as a way to boost their economies and make it possible for digital technologies to take off. They see their job as making it possible, by building the necessary structure, for private companies to provide content to improve health care, education, and communications. Political leaders in these places have not waited on the market to wire their nation; instead they use the public sector to build infrastructure and trust that private companies will provide relevant content.

Countries such as South Korea, Taiwan, and Singapore have superfast networks for information technology. People can access digital information through computers, cell phones, or handheld devices. Some of these nations have "smart cards" that allow people to complete online transactions with great confidence regarding their personal privacy and security. These countries justify the infrastructure costs as an investment in their future economic development.

Other nations, such as the United States, have lagged behind in building broadband infrastructure. In contrast to many others, the U.S. government has felt that private companies, not the public sector, should fund the development of broadband infrastructure and has left it to the private sector to implement. As a result, places that lack the income or population density required to justify commercial investments lag behind; while dense urban and suburban areas get wired for digital access, rural and poor neighborhoods do not. That creates a patchwork of Internet and cell phone connections that inhibits communications and makes it difficult to build reliable networks over broad geographical areas.

Under such circumstances, mobile phone companies drop calls and in some places it is impossible to get an Internet connection. Rather than there being a nationwide network of digital and wireless broadband, there is a marble cake of different designs, connections, and bandwidth, making it difficult to create a reliable network on which consumers and businesses can depend for commerce, entertainment, and social networking.

If public officials want electronic health services to flourish, they must budget the funds and build the political coalitions necessary to promote investment in the required technologies. Modern societies require highspeed communication networks, and governments play a crucial role in building those networks. Without public sector involvement, digital medicine will not generate the desired service improvements and necessary cost savings.

The United States is to join the rest of the developed world by 2011 in moving from the World Health Organization's International Classification of Diseases (ICD) level 9 to level 10. The ICD system is employed across nations to track health care and classify specific diseases and treatments. Level 10 was adopted by France and the United Kingdom in 1995; by Germany, Australia, and Brazil in 1998; and by Russia in 1999, Canada in 2001, and China in 2002.[27]

When the United States migrates to this standard, it will provide an opportunity to upgrade health information systems and develop more sophisticated digital processes. In much the way that the Y2K deadline forced governments, businesses, and organizations to update their computer systems at the turn of the twenty-first century, ICD-10 will prod health providers to think systematically about health information technology and how to employ broadband communications to save money and improve operating efficiency. Deadlines often help policymakers to move forward with needed policy innovations, and this milestone provides an opportunity for digital medicine advocates to insist on infrastructure development.

Some progress already is being seen on advanced technology usage facilitated by high-speed broadband. The McKesson Corporation, for example, has developed what it calls an "all-digital hospital." Methodist Hospital in Dublin, Ohio, features computerized doctor order entry systems, scanning of patients' bar-coded wrist bands to match patient and medication dosages, digital scheduling of health professionals, electronic medical records, and remote X-ray imaging.[28]

The Cerner Corporation has unveiled what it labels the hospital "Smart Room": an all-computerized treatment facility in which all the medical devices are linked to the patient's electronic medical record. The facility also includes interactive television, laptop computers, video conferencing capability for external medical consultations, and a medical dashboard that displays up-to-date medical history and treatments.[29] Cerner also has implemented "health homes" that integrate patients' medical records with treatment plans, payment systems, and health monitoring devices that alert health care providers when changes in blood pressure, heart rate, or weight warrant new treatment options.

TRAINING MEDICAL PROFESSIONALS

It is important to focus not just on consumer education and infrastructure development but also on training health care providers about the utility of health information technology. If savings are to be gained from the use of digital medical resources, doctors and nurses must be informed about its benefits and costs and trained to make the transition from paper to electronic recordkeeping systems.[30] Only if that happens will they be able to implement new digital systems and benefit from them.

Some observers already worry about the quality of medical care with the advent of high-tech instruments. Patients like the convenience of making appointments and renewing prescriptions online, but they are concerned about whether health treatments will be as good and effective as they have come to expect with in-person care.[31] Of course, even primary care physicians are not able to spend as much time with patients as patients would like, but even short personal encounters provide an opportunity for spontaneous questions that can yield valuable treatment information.

Health care providers must understand that as a medical experience, digital encounters differ significantly from personal contact. They must allow time for questions and structure electronic interactions in order to facilitate quality patient care. Merely assuming that the two settings allow for similar types of caregiving will not produce the improvements desired by consumers. Digital interactions must be adapted to the needs of people accustomed to personalized health care. If consumers do not obtain the individualized care that they want, digital medicine will not reach the desired policy goals.

Policymakers hope that a major portion of U.S. patients will use electronic medical records by 2014.[32] That ambitious deadline was set to make sure that usage increases enough that doctors are willing to invest the necessary resources in digital communications and that the health care system becomes more efficient and effective at caregiving. The public must embrace technology if health care providers are to reap the economies of scale possible through increased expenditures on technology.

However, cost remains a major barrier to the adoption of new technology. According to a study of electronic medical records in primary care, installation of electronic records cost $13,100 per provider per year, including software, hardware, support services, and maintenance. That would bring the total expenditure over a five-year period to $46,400. Benefits in terms of savings on transcription, billing, and administration were estimated at $5,700 in year 1; $24,300 in year 2; $24,300 in year 3; $50,300 in year 4; and $50,300 in year 5, for a five-year total of $154,900. That results in a net benefit of $108,500 with a present value of $86,400.[33]

Training is important with these systems because surveys indicate that initially medical professionals find them difficult to use. Most professional systems have multiple screens, various options, and a variety of navigational approaches.[34] Learning to use these systems involves a considerable investment of time up front, with the payoff coming several years down the road. In an industry with extensive time and cost pressures, such barriers make it difficult to implement this kind of improvement.

One case study of an internal medicine practice that implemented electronic medical records found that both personal and financial costs were quite high. The total cost of the system was $140,000. Both staff and doctors had to undergo extensive training on data entry and system maintenance. Midway through implementation, the system was attacked by a virus, which led to an extensive drain on staff time. Moving to the electronic system required a redesign of office work flow and daily routines. Although all providers concluded that the transition was worthwhile, the doctors felt that small medical offices would not be able to adopt an electronic system unless financial assistance was provided. Their view was that a subsidy of at least $12,000 per physician per year would be required to convince recalcitrant doctors to move in this direction.[35]

One of the obstacles to the adoption of new systems is the absence of common technical standards for electronic medical records.[36] Each health practice has to choose its own software and hardware configuration from many different sources, and it is difficult to know which is the best. No one wants to invest money in a system if it cannot communicate with those of other providers. Interoperability, or the ability of technology systems to communicate with one another, is a major problem. When health care providers use different hardware and software systems, communicating across different platforms is a challenge. It slows the pace of innovation, and it is costly and frustrating for all involved.[37]

Some states have solved the problem of lack of uniform standards by letting a dominant local player dictate the market. In Tennessee, for example, Governor Phil Breeden approved comprehensive health care reform to control pharmacy spending, limit personal health benefits, and provide for health insurance cost sharing with employees. Vanderbilt University developed a quality information system that integrated existing office systems of local medical professionals on an incremental basis, giving them excellent interoperability with regional systems. That simplified the choice for local medical professionals because many of them were able to adopt the same recordkeeping system.[38]

Some writers have called for improved federal support for health information systems. In recent years, the national government has provided subsidies for new systems, but primarily in the area of billing, not medical records. That has limited the ability of the industry to move ahead while highlighting the importance of the federal role in technological innovation. In effect, a two-tiered system has emerged in which larger practices have the resources to invest in technology while smaller practices do not. Federal officials could have a very positive effect by writing uniform standards, providing financial support, and promoting interoperability of technical systems.[39]

The federal government has provided new incentives for doctors to adopt electronic medical records. In 2008, the Medicare program announced a trial program in which providers who move from paper to electronic recordkeeping will receive higher Medicare payments to compensate for the extra time that they take to complete online prescriptions or enter test results.[40] Individual physicians will receive up to $58,000 over five years to participate in the program. Those who have joined the program feel it has improved the quality of health care and helped them avoid treatment or prescription errors.[41]

Some employers and health insurers are providing doctors with financial incentives to provide e-mail consultations and mechanisms for electronic prescription orders. At the request of the nonprofit National Committee for Quality Assurance, medical professionals are receiving higher reimbursements from health insurers for spending more time with patients and providing high-quality health care. Boeing, for example, has undertaken a pilot program to provide doctors with financial incentives for e-mail consultations that has gotten positive feedback from doctors and patients alike.[42]

However, critics claim that the market will not solve the problems that limit the use of health information technology unless the U.S. federal government takes a more active role in supporting technological innovation. Market forces fragment the medical system and thereby accentuate interoperability problems. Private businesses simply do not have an incentive to develop uniform types of technology. They make money by selling different systems that are not based on uniform technical standards, and that will not change unless federal officials mandate more uniform standards.[43]

The other option for electronic health records is for patients to take responsibility for their own records rather than rely on doctors or hospitals. Microsoft has an Internet initiative called HealthVault, which, in partnership with McKesson Corporation's RelayHealth, allows individuals to place their personal medical records online at a secure and encrypted website.[44] Users determine what health information to put on the site and who has access. They can give visitors one-time or ongoing access privileges, allowing them to control who sees what part of their medical records.[45] Through RelayHealth, doctors can order prescriptions electronically and store information in the patient's electronic medical record.

Not only can consumers store their own records online, the site allows users to upload data from home diagnostic and other kinds of devices to HealthVault, where the data can be accessed by either the consumer or specified health care providers. For example, data regarding heart rate, power, and GPS locations can be uploaded to this website. Among the organizations that have signed up for HealthVault are the Mayo Clinic, the American Heart Association, MedStar, LifeScan, and various hospitals around the country.[46]

In order to pay for the service, Microsoft relies on advertisements connected to its search engine. Visitors can request information about grouped topics such as nutrition, medication, and clinical research. That allows advertisers to target particular searches and place sponsored links next to the search results. Microsoft expects an advertising market of between $500 million to $1 billion that will grow to $5 billion within seven years. Referring to the increase in the online advertising market, Peter Neupert, the Microsoft executive in charge of this site, said "It's all about search."[47]

However, some scientists complain about possible threats to the confidentiality of patient records because organizations such as Microsoft and Google are not subject to the privacy rules of the Health Insurance Portability and Accountability Act (HIPAA). Conventional medical providers such as doctors, nurses, and hospitals face strict regulations regarding what health information they can share with other professionals.[48] Commercial information technology companies, however, are not subject to the same requirements.

Moreover, heavy reliance on commercial advertising at websites that offer online storage of medical records creates potential conflict-of-interest problems for consumers who use them. Consumers seeking impartial material may not realize that particular links are sponsored by self-interested advertisers and may have difficulty distinguishing for-profit from nonprofit sources of information. That hurts the credibility of online health information and may slow the adoption of electronic medical records by consumers who already are skeptical of online resources.

OVERCOMING LEGAL AND POLITICAL OBSTACLES

Perhaps the toughest problem for digital medicine is not technology, but politics and law. The health care system is highly fragmented, and a wide variety of powerful political actors have divergent interests in it.[49] The interests of hospitals, doctors, insurers, pharmaceutical companies, lawyers, and patients are not the same, and it therefore is difficult to build coalitions that allow the health care system to move forward. In the electronic medical records area, for example, health care providers argue about who should have control of the records: patients, doctors, hospitals, or insurance companies. Until that dispute is resolved, adoption of electronic records will not progress at a very rapid pace.[50]

If digital medicine is to flourish, political leaders must decide what kind of reimbursement rates should be available for e-mail consultations, digital prescriptions, and other electronic health services. Right now, only twenty-three of the fifty states allow digital prescriptions.[51] E-health and telecare rates vary considerably by jurisdiction, and the hodge-podge of regulations and reimbursement schedules makes it difficult for doctors to know how to proceed with new technologies. If there is reimbursement for office visits but not e-mail consultations, medical professionals are going to discourage patients from contacting them by e-mail.

Many health insurers do not provide any reimbursement for electronic consultations; consequently, many doctors are working for free when they answer patient e-mails. However, under one proposal, patients would pay a flat rate ranging from $100 to several hundred dollars a year for e-mail consultations. A research team found that with this type of consultation, "doctors and patients move closer together, and trust grows strikingly. Interchange becomes more personal, and office visits seem more efficient and less emotionally charged."[52]

Other doctors feel that they cannot answer patient e-mails without violating HIPAA, which guarantees the confidentiality of patients' medical records; therefore, they forbid answering e-mail through conventional devices because they cannot safeguard the confidentiality of a reply outside the office's firewall. Clearly, this problem needs to be resolved in order to facilitate the emergence of digital medicine.

Physicians interested in digital medicine have found four services to be popular: online appointments, prescription refills, consultations, and messaging. Some practices have reported a nearly 20 percent drop in the number of phone calls when web messaging is added, allowing patients to make appointments and order refills through the Internet.[53] It is clear that the opportunity to improve productivity through technology requires solutions to delicate legal and political matters.

TAKING ETHICS AND PRIVACY SERIOUSLY

The final obstacle limiting digital medicine concerns ethics and privacy. Public opinion surveys indicate that ordinary people worry about the confidentiality of online transactions and conflicts of interest within the medical profession. Indeed, one of the most important barriers to increased use of electronic health resources cited in consumer polls is privacy concerns. According to poll data, 39 percent of people name insufficient privacy of the Internet as their top worry about health information technology.[54]

The age group most concerned about invasion of privacy is young people. They periodically search for sensitive health care information online but worry whether their searches will remain confidential; they want to make sure that parents, employers, and insurance companies do not find out. According to health researchers, that concern often makes them less likely to employ the Internet for health information.[55]

Mistrust is ironic in the case of young people because they are the age group most likely to use the Internet and other digital resources in general. They love the convenience and accessibility of electronic resources and its around-the-clock availability. Young adults often spend a substantial part of their day using online communications and visiting social networking websites.

However, if worry about ethics and privacy restrains the usage of health information technology, it becomes a serious barrier to increased use of digital medical resources. All users must feel confident about the security of their information if they are to make use of the new opportunities for online communication.

CONCLUSION

There is little doubt that in the short run, there will continue to be major barriers to digital medicine. Concerns over privacy, confidentiality, trustworthiness, and cost limit the ability of electronic resources to achieve the gains in efficiency, effectiveness, and quality desired by health technology advocates. Usage must increase much more in order for there to be any hope of attaining economies of scale. Policymakers must understand the importance of concrete action on those problems to improve public confidence in needed reforms.

In the long run, however, progress will be made on many of the current policy challenges. Health care cost projections virtually guarantee that policy innovations will be introduced and problems that slow progression now will be overcome. Health care costs are escalating so rapidly that policymakers have little choice but to take meaningful action. Failure to act is no longer an option.

Nearly every major political leader in the United States sees digital medicine as a necessary reform that will improve quality, reduce costs, and extend access to more and more people. Politicians as different as Newt Gingrich, Barack Obama, and Hillary Clinton have embraced health information technology.[56] While this study demonstrates the limits to optimism, there is no question that there is agreement across the political spectrum on the importance of innovation in health care technology.

The only question concerns how fast new measures will unfold and in what form. The e-health revolution is here. It clearly will take financial investment and political action to speed up the revolution and achieve the desired results. If public policymakers are able to educate consumers, train medical providers, and close the digital divide, they will extend the benefits of digital medicine to more people.

Appendixes

A. NATIONAL E-HEALTH PUBLIC OPINION SURVEY

Survey Methods

From November 5 to November 10, 2005, we undertook a national survey of 1,428 adults aged 18 and older in the continental forty-eight states. Trained and paid interviewers at the John Hazen White Sr. Public Opinion Laboratory at Brown University asked respondents about forms of health communication, satisfaction with health services, knowledge levels, health status, and lifestyle behaviors. We also collected basic information such as age, gender, race, insurance status, education level, residence, income, and perceived health. The margin of error in this survey was ± 3 percentage points, assuming simple random sampling. We placed up to three callbacks to reach respondents.

The sample was provided to the authors by a commercial sampling firm, Survey Sampling, Inc. It was based on a randomly generated set of telephone numbers stratified by state to ensure proper geographic representation. It had also undergone prior screening using automated methods to ensure inclusion of working numbers. The initial sampling frame included 5,000 telephone numbers, approximately three-quarters of which were households and therefore were eligible for inclusion in the survey. Of the 3,725 eligible households, 1,428 answered the telephone, providing us with a contact rate of 38.3 percent, including 500 who refused to participate and 928 who completed the survey. Thus, we received responses from approximately 25.0 percent of all eligible households (928 of 3,725) and 65.0 percent of households contacted (928 of 1,428), with the former being the *response rate* and the latter the *cooperation rate*, according to American Association for Public Opinion Research definitions.

Survey Questions

"Hello, I'm calling from the Center for Public Policy at Brown University. We are conducting a study of people's opinions about health care and we'd really appreciate your help. I'd like to ask a few questions of the youngest male, 18 years of age or older, who is now at home." (If not available, speak to oldest female, 18 years of age or older, now at home.)

State Abbreviation: ___

Code gender of respondent: 1: male, 2: female, 9: don't know.

In the past year, how often did you visit a doctor or other health care provider? 1: not at all, 2: once every few months, 3: once a month, 4: once a week, 8: don't know, 9: no answer.

In the past year, how often did you visit an emergency room? 1: not at all, 2: once every few months, 3: once a month, 4: once a week, 8: don't know, 9: no answer.

In the past year, how often did you telephone a doctor or other health care provider for medical or treatment advice? 1: not at all, 2: once every few months, 3: once a month, 4: once a week, 8: don't know, 9: no answer.

In the past year, how often did you use e-mail to communicate with a doctor or other health care provider? 1: not at all, 2: once every few months, 3: once a month, 4: once a week, 8: don't know, 9: no answer.

In the past year, how often did you use e-mail or the Internet to communicate with other people who have health conditions or concerns like you? 1: not at all, 2: once every few months, 3: once a month, 4: once a week, 8: don't know, 9: no answer.

In the past year, how often did you use e-mail or the Internet to purchase a prescription drug? 1: not at all, 2: once every few months, 3: once a month, 4: once a week, 8: don't know, 9: no answer.

In the past year, how often did you use e-mail or the Internet to purchase medical equipment or devices? 1: not at all, 2: once every few months, 3: once a month, 4: once a week, 8: don't know, 9: no answer.

In the past year, how often did you look on commercial Internet websites for information about health care? 1: not at all 2: once every few months 3: once a month 4: once a week 8: don't know 9: no answer

In the past year, how often did you look on nonprofit Internet websites for information about health care? 1: not at all, 2: once every few months, 3: once a month, 4: once a week, 8: don't know, 9: no answer.

In the past year, how often did you visit government health department websites for information about health care? 1: not at all, 2: once every few months, 3: once a month, 4: once a week, 8: don't know, 9: no answer.

Do you have electronic medical records that store details of your health condition? 1: yes, 2: no, 8: don't know, 9: no answer.

Overall, how would you rate your current health? 1: excellent, 2: very good, 3: good, 4: fair, 5: poor, 6: very poor, 8: don't know, 9: no answer.

How often do you exercise? 1: not at all, 2: once every few months, 3: once a month, 4: once a week, 5: once a day, 8: don't know, 9: no answer.

How often do you eat a balanced diet? 1: not at all, 2: once every few months, 3: once a month, 4: once a week, 5: once a day, 6: every meal, 8: don't know, 9: no answer.

How often do you smoke? 1: not at all, 2: once every few months, 3: once a month, 4: once a week, 5: once a day, 6: several times a day, 8: don't know, 9: no answer.

How often do you have someone help you read medical materials? 1: always, 2: often, 3: sometimes, 4: occasionally, 5: never, 8: don't know, 9: no answer.

How confident are you filling out medical forms by yourself? 1: always, 2: often, 3: sometimes, 4: occasionally, 5: never, 8: don't know, 9: no answer.

How often do you have problems learning about your medical condition because of difficulty understanding written information? 1: always, 2: often, 3: sometimes, 4: occasionally, 5: never, 8: don't know, 9: no answer.

Overall, would you rate the quality of the American health care system as: 1: excellent, 2: very good, 3: good, 4: fair, 5: poor, or 6: very poor? 8: don't know, 9: no answer.

How strongly do you agree or disagree with each of the following statements?

a. I think my doctor's office has everything needed to provide complete medical care: 1: strongly agree, 2: agree, 3: uncertain, 4: disagree, 5: strongly disagree, 9: no answer.

b. Sometimes doctors make me wonder if their diagnosis is correct: 1: strongly agree, 2: agree, 3: uncertain, 4: disagree, 5: strongly disagree, 9: no answer.

c. When I go for medical care, they are careful to check everything when treating and examining me: 1: strongly agree, 2: agree, 3: uncertain, 4: disagree, 5: strongly disagree, 9: no answer.

d. Doctors act too businesslike and impersonal toward me: 1: strongly agree, 2: agree, 3: uncertain, 4: disagree, 5: strongly disagree, 9: no answer.

e. Those who provide my medical care sometimes hurry too much when they treat me: 1: strongly agree, 2: agree, 3: uncertain, 4: disagree, 5: strongly disagree, 9: no answer.

f. I find it hard to get an appointment for medical care right away: 1: strongly agree, 2: agree, 3: uncertain, 4: disagree, 5: strongly disagree, 9: no answer.

g. I am able to get medical care whenever I need it: 1: strongly agree, 2: agree, 3: uncertain, 4: disagree, 5: strongly disagree, 9: no answer.

How worried are you about whether you can afford the health care that you and your family need? 1: very worried, 2: somewhat worried, 3: not very worried, 8: don't know, 9: no answer.

In the past year, have you or a family member had any problems paying medical bills? 1: yes, 2: no, 8: don't know, 9: no answer.

Do you currently have health insurance? 1: yes, 2: no, 8: don't know, 9: no answer.

Regardless of how you vote, do you usually think of yourself as a Republican, a Democrat, an Independent, or something else? 1: Republican, 2: Democrat, 3: Independent, 4: Other, 9: no answer.

Do you consider yourself a: 1: conservative, 2: moderate, or 3: liberal? 8: don't know, 9: no answer.

Which of the following age groups are you in? 1: 18–24, 2: 25–34, 3: 35–44, 4: 45–54, 5: 55–64, 6: 65–74, 7: 75–84, 8: 85 or older, 9: no answer.

Is your overall family income: 1: $0–$15,000, 2: $15,001–$30,000, 3: $30,001–$50,000, 4: $50,001–$75,000, 5: $75,001–$100,000, 6: $100,001–$150,000, 7: over $150,000? 8: don't know, 9: no answer.

What is the highest grade of school you have completed? 1: 0–8 years, 2: some high school, 3: high school graduate, 4: some college, 5: college graduate, 6: postgraduate work, 8: don't know, 9: no answer.

Do you live in a: 1: rural, 2: suburban, or 3: urban area? 8: don't know, 9: no answer.

Are you: 1: nonwhite Hispanic, 2: African American, 3: Hispanic, 4: Asian American, or 5: something else? 8: don't know, 9: no answer.

(If respondent is not sure or names more than one group) Would you say you feel closest to being: 1: nonwhite Hispanic, 2: African American, 3: Hispanic, 4: Asian American, or 5: something else? 8: don't know, 9: no answer.

B. AMERICAN HEALTH WEBSITES

A. Most Popular Commercial Websites

(as determined by Nielsen/NetRatings)
1. US Fitness—www.usfitness.com
2. WebMD—www.webmd.com
3. Drugstore.com—www.drugstore.com
4. Walgreens.com—www.walgreens.com
5. Yahoo!Health—http://health.yahoo.com
6. About.com Health—www.about.com/health
7. MSN Health & Fitness—http://health.msn.com
8. AOL Health—http://body.aol.com/health
9. MedicineNet.com—www.medicinenet.com
10. Medco—www.medco.com
11. Everyday Health Network—www.everydayhealth.com

12. Quality Health—www.qualityhealth.com/psp/homepage.jspa
13. Weight Watchers—www.weightwatchers.com/index.aspx
14. Real Age—www.realage.com/homepage.aspx
15. Drugs.com—www.drugs.com
16. CVS Pharmacy—www.cvs.com
17. Aetna—www.aetna.com/index.htm
18. LifeScript—www.lifescript.com
19. MyUHC.com—www.myuhc.com
20. RX List—www.rxlist.com/script/main/hp.asp
21. HealthLine—www.healthline.com
22. ThatsFit—www.thatsfit.com
23. eMedicine.com—www.emedicine.com
24. Prevention—www.prevention.com/cda/homepage.do
25. AmbienCR—www.ambiencr.com
26. Healthology—www.healthology.com
27. eDiets—www.ediets.com
28. ExpressScripts.com—www.expressscripts.com
29. eMedicineHealth—www.emedicinehealth.com/script/main/hp.asp
30. Lime Health Blog—www.lime.com
31. Medscape—www.medscape.com/home
32. HealthGrades—www.healthgrades.com
33. Nutrisystem—www.nutrisystem.com
34. Pfizer—www.pfizer.com/pfizer/main.jsp
35. Blue Cross Blue Shield Association—www.bluecrossblueshield.com
36. iVillage Health and Fitness—http://health.ivillage.com
37. Rite Aid—www.riteaid.com
38. The Biggest Loser Club—www2.biggestloserclub.com
39. Care Pages.com—www.carepages.com
40. HealthcareSource—www.healthcaresource.com
41. Mercola.com—www.mercola.com
42. HealthSquare—www.healthsquare.com
43. Chantix—www.chantix.com
44. NetDoctor—www.netdoctor.co.uk

B. Top Nonprofit Websites

(as determined by the Medical Library Association's Consumer and Patient Health Information Section)

1. The Mayo Clinic—www.themayoclinic.com
2. Kid's Health—www.kidshealth.org

3. FamilyDoctor.org—http://familydoctor.org/online/famdocen/home.html
4. MedHelp—www.medhelp.org
5. HealthLink Plus—www.healthlinkplus.org
6. Hardin MD—www.lib.uiowa.edu/hardin/md
7. Net Wellness—www.netwellness.org
8. The Cleveland Clinic—www.clevelandclinic.org
9. NOAH Health—www.noah-health.org
10. National Women's Health Resource Center—www.healthywomen.org
11. Our Bodies Ourselves—www.ourbodiesourselves.org
12. The North American Menopause Society—www.menopause.org/default.htm
13. American Urological Association—www.urologyhealth.org
14. American Academy of Pediatrics—www.aap.org
15. The Virtual Pediatric Hospital—www.virtualpediatrichospital.org
16. The American Geriatric Society Foundation for Health in Aging—www.healthinaging.org
17. The Family Caregiver Alliance—www.caregiver.org/caregiver/jsp/home.jsp
18. The Alzheimer's Association—www.alz.org
19. The American Academy of Dermatology—www.aad.org/default.htm
20. The American Dental Association—www.ada.org
21. The American Diabetes Association—www.diabetes.org/home.jsp
22. The American Heart Association—www.americanheart.org/presenter.jhtml?identifier=1200000
23. The American Lung Association—www.lungusa.org/site/pp.asp?c=dvLUK9O0E&b=22542
24. The Asthma and Allergy Foundation—www.aafa.org/index.cfm
25. American Academy of Orthopaedic Surgeons—www.aaos.org
26. Memorial Sloan Kettering Cancer Center—www.mskcc.org/mskcc/html/1979.cfm
27. HealthWeb—www.healthweb.org
28. The Public Library of Science—www.plos.org
29. American Medical Association Doctor Finder—http://webapps.ama-assn.org/doctorfinder/home.jsp
30. HighWire Press—http://highwire.stanford.edu

C. State Government Health Websites

Alabama: "Department of Public Health"—www.adph.org
Alaska: "Health and Social Services"—www.hss.state.ak.us

Arizona: "Department of Health Services"—www.azdhs.gov

Arkansas: "Arkansas Department of Health"—www.healthyarkansas.com

California: "Health"—www.ca.gov/Health.html

Colorado: "Department of Public Health and Environment"—
www.cdphe.state.co.us

Connecticut: "Department of Public Health"—www.dph.state.ct.us

Delaware: "Health and Human Services"—
www.dhss.delaware.gov/dhss/index.html

Florida: "Department of Health"—www.doh.state.fl.us

Georgia: "Family and Health"—www.georgia.gov/00/channel_title/
0,2094,4802_4965,00.html

Hawaii: "State Department of Health"—http://www.hawaii.gov/health

Idaho: "Department of Health and Welfare"—www.healthandwelfare.
idaho.gov

Illinois: "Health and Wellness"—http://health.illinois.gov

Indiana: "State Department of Health"—www.in.gov/isdh

Iowa: "Department of Public Health"—www.idph.state.ia.us

Kansas: "State Department of Health and Environment, Division of
Health"—www.kdheks.gov/health/index.html

Kentucky: "Department of Public Health"—http://chfs.ky.gov/dph/
default.htm

Louisiana: "Department of Health and Hospitals"—www.dhh.
louisiana.gov

Maine: "Department of Health and Human Services"—www.maine.
gov/dhhs

Maryland: "Department of Health and Mental Hygiene"—
www.dhmh.state.md.us

Massachusetts: "Department of Public Health"—www.mass.gov/dph

Michigan: "Health"—www.michigan.gov/som/0,1607,7-192-29942—
-,00.html

Minnesota: "Department of Health"—www.health.state.mn.us/
index.html

Mississippi: "State Department of Health"—www.msdh.state.ms.us

Missouri: "Department of State and Senior Services"—www.dhss.mo.gov

Montana: "Department of Public Health and Human Services"—
www.dphhs.mt.gov

Nebraska: "Department of Health and Human Services"—www.hhs.
state.ne.us

Nevada: "Department of Health and Human Services, Health
Division"—http://health2k.state.nv.us

New Hampshire: "Department of Health and Human Services"—
www.dhhs.nh.gov/DHHS/DHHS_SITE/default.htm

New Jersey: "Department of Health and Senior Services"—www.state.
nj.us/health

New Mexico: "Health Department"—www.health.state.nm.us

New York: "Department of Health"—www.health.state.ny.us

North Carolina: "Department of Health and Human Services"—
www.ncdhhs.gov/health/index.htm

North Dakota: "Department of Health"—www.health.state.nd.us

Ohio: "Department of Health"—www.odh.ohio.gov

Oklahoma: "State Department of Health"—www.health.state.ok.us

Oregon: "Department of Human Services"—www.oregon.gov/DHS/
index.shtml

Pennsylvania: "Department of Health"—www.dsf.health.state.pa.us

Rhode Island: "Department of Health"—www.health.ri.gov

South Carolina: "Department of Health and Human Services"—
www.dhhs.state.sc.us/dhhsnew/index.asp

South Dakota: "Department of Health"—http://doh.sd.gov

Tennessee: "Department of Health"—http://health.state.tn.us/index.shtml

Texas: "Department of State Health Services"—www.dshs.state.tx.us

Utah: "Department of Health"—www.health.utah.gov

Vermont: "Department of Health"—http://healthvermont.gov

Virginia: "Department of Health"—www.vdh.state.va.us/index.htm

Washington: "State Department of Health"—www.doh.wa.gov

West Virginia: "Bureau for Public Health"—www.wvdhhr.org/bph

Wisconsin: "Department of Health and Family Services"—
www.dhfs.state.wi.us

Wyoming: "Department of Health"—http://wdh.state.wy.us

C. GOVERNMENT HEALTH DEPARTMENT WEBSITES AROUND THE WORLD

Algeria: "Ministry of Health"—www.ands.dz

Argentina: "Ministerio de Salud"—www.msal.gov.ar/htm/default.asp

Arab Emirates: "Ministry of Health"—www.moh.gov.ae/intro

Australia: "Department of Health and Aging"—www.health.gov.au

Bahrain: "Ministry of Health"—www.moh.gov.bh/index.asp

Belgium: "Ministry of Public Health"—www.health.fgov.be

Brazil: "Ministerio de Saude"—http://portal.saude.gov.br/saude

Canada: "Health Canada"—www.hc-sc.gc.ca/index_e.html

Chile: "Ministerio de Salud"—www.minsal.cl

China: "Ministry of Health"—www.moh.gov.cn

Cuba: "Ministry of Public Health"—www.dne.sld.cu/minsap/index.htm

Denmark: "Ministry of the Interior and Health"—www.im.dk/im

El Salvador: "Ministerio de Salud"—www.mspas.gob.sv

Estonia: "Ministry of Social Affairs: Public Health"—www.sm.ee/eng/
pages/index.html

Fiji: "Ministry of Health"—www.fiji.gov.fj/publish/m_health.shtml

Finland: "National Public Health Institute"—www.ktl.fi/portal/English

France: "Ministère de la Santé"—www.sante.gouv.fr

Germany: "Ministry of Health"—www.bmg.bund.de/cln_041/nn_
617002/EN/Health/health-node,param=.html__nnn=true

Great Britain: "Health and Wellbeing"—www.direct.gov.uk/en/
HealthAndWellBeing/index.htm

Hong Kong: "Department of Health"—www.dh.gov.hk/index.htm

Hungary: "Ministry of Health"—www.eum.hu

Iceland: "Ministry of Health and Social Security"—http://eng.
heilbrigdisraduneyti.is

India: "Ministry of Health and Family Welfare"—http://mohfw.nic.in

Iran: "Ministry of Health and Medical Information"—www.mohme.
gov.ir/FFolder/web.aspx

Iraq: www.iraqigovernment.org

Ireland: "Department of Health and Children"—www.dohc.ie

Israel: "Ministry of Health"—www.health.gov.il

Jamaica: "Ministry of Health"—www.moh.gov.jm

Japan: "Ministry of Health, Labour and Welfare"—www.mhlw.go.jp/
english/index.html

Kenya: "Ministry of Health"—www.health.go.ke

Kuwait: "Ministry of Health"—www.moh.gov.kw

Lebanon: "Ministry of Public Health"—www.public-health.gov.lb

Lesotho: "Ministry of Health and Social Welfare"—www.lesotho.gov.
ls/health

Luxembourg: "Ministère de la Santé"—www.ms.etat.lu

Malaysia: "Department of Public Health"—www.dph.gov.my

Maldives: "Health"—www.maldivesinfo.gov.mv/info/include/
health_health_status.php

Malta: "Ministry for Health, the Elderly, and Community Care"—
www.ehealth.gov.mt

Mexico: "Secretaría de Salud"—http://portal.salud.gob.mx

Mauritius: "Ministry of Health and the Quality of Life"—www.gov.
mu/portal/site/mohsite

New Zealand: "Ministry of Health"—www.moh.govt.nz/moh.nsf

Norway: "Ministry of Health and Care Services"—www.regjeringen.
no/en/dep/hod.html?id=421

Nicaragua: "Ministerio de Salud"—www.minsa.gob.ni

Panama: "Ministerio de Salud"—www.minsa.gob.pa

Paraguay: "Ministerio de Salud Publica"—www.mspbs.gov.py

Peru: "Ministerio de Salud"—www.minsa.gob.pe/portal

Philippines: "Department of Health"—www.doh.gov.ph

Poland: "Ministry of Health and Social Security"—www.mzios.gov.pl

Qatar: "Ministry of Health"—www.hmc.org.qa/hmc/mph_a/default.htm

Saudi Arabia: "Ministry of Health"—www.moh.gov.sa/ar/index.php

Sénégal: "Ministère de la Santé et de la Prévention Médicale"—
www.sante.gouv.sn

Singapore: "Ministry of Health"—www.moh.gov.sg

Slovenia: "Ministry of Health"—www.mz.gov.si/en

South Africa: "Department of Health"—www.doh.gov.za

South Korea: "Ministry of Health and Welfare"—http://english.mohw.
go.kr/index.jsp

Spain: "Ministerio de Sanidad y Consumo"—www.msc.es/en/home.htm

Sweden: "Ministry of Health and Social Affairs"—www.sweden.gov.se/
sb/d/2061

Switzerland: "Federal Office of Public Health"—www.bag.admin.ch/
index.html?lang=en

Syria: "Ministry of Health"—www.moh.gov.sy

Taiwan: "Department of Health"—www.doh.gov.tw/dohenglish

Tanzania: "Ministry of Health"—www.tanzania.go.tz/health.htm

Thailand: "Ministry of Public Health"—http://eng.moph.go.th

Turkey: "The Ministry of Health of Turkey"—www.saglik.gov.tr/EN/
Default.aspx?17A16AE30572D313AAF6AA849816B2EF4376734B
ED947CDE

Ukraine: "Ministry of Health"—www.health.gov.ua

United States: "Department of Health and Human Services"—
www.hhs.gov

Vietnam: "Ministry of Health"—www.moh.gov.vn/homebyt/vn/
portal/index.jsp

Zimbabwe: "Ministry of Health and Child Welfare"—www.mohcw.gov.zw

D. CONTENT ANALYSIS PROTOCOL FOR HEALTH CARE WEBSITES

Website name: such as Human Services. The name of the website can be shortened down (that is, just typing "agriculture" instead of "department of agriculture"). However, it is very helpful to use the complete name of the website name in case you have to go back to a site you previously worked on.

Has online publications: 0: no, 1: yes. This category includes news releases, newsletters, journals, reports, studies, laws, or constitutions. Often, major reports are in PDF format, and these would count as publications as well.

Offers online databases: 0: no, 1: yes. This can range widely from statistics, charts, tables, and data to actual databases (which are like search engines except that they are customized to retrieve specific information rather than search the entire website). Databases are often found in the statistics, information, or publications sections of webpages. However, phone directories and job opening listings do not count as a database.

Has audio clips: 0: no, 1: yes. Any sound file whatsoever, whether it be in the form of a speech; radio show; radio public service announcement; podcast; or a website welcome or music, such as a state song or national anthem. These can often be deeply embedded in websites and hard to find. Try searching Google for "site: www.site.gov audio." Also try other Google searches that might turn up audio files by replacing "audio" with "mp3," "windows media player," or "real player."

Has video clips: 0: no, 1: yes. Any video file. Examples are televised speeches and events, department commercials, public service announcements, and website welcome. Could be a video clip or example of streaming video. These can often be deeply embedded in websites and hard to find. Try searching Google for "site: www.site.gov video." Also try other Google searches that might turn up audio files by replacing "video" with "mpg," "windows media player," "real player." Power-Point presentations, slideshows, and Java content are not included as video clips. Some sites display noncontinuous webcam images (for example, a traffic webcam, which updates every 5 seconds)—these do not count as video clips either.

Has foreign language or language translation: 0: no, 1: yes. Can be a webpage entirely in a non-native language (for example, a webpage translated into Español for English-speaking countries), a link to language translating software like Babel Fish, or publications available in other languages. Some sites have links to translation software from the home page. Other sites have only a publication (for example, a driver's manual) or a downloadable form in another language—this counts. As these can be hard to find, try searching Google for "site: www.site.gov espanol" or "site: www.site.gov Spanish."

Has commercial ads: 0: no, 1: yes. Do not count as ads those links to website developer and computer software available for free download, such as Adobe Acrobat Reader, Netscape Navigator, or Microsoft Internet Explorer, since they are necessary for viewing pages. Traditional banner or pop-up ads that the advertiser paid for count. Ads have to be clear commercial sponsorships of a product or service. It must appear that the advertiser paid for the placement and that the ad must lead the visitor to the external commercial website. Listings of phone numbers and web addresses provided for the visitor's convenience (such as a directory of airlines or hotels or a listing of tax assistance services) do not count. In our study, many links on sites appeared to be ads, but after clicking on them, they were only promoting a particular government program or event. Links promoting state tourism often took this form.

Has a website section requiring a premium fee for entry: 0: no, 1: yes. Fee required to access particular areas on website (such as business services, access to databases, or viewing of up-to-the-minute legislation). This is not the same as a user fee for a single service. For example, some government services require payment to complete the transaction; that does not count. This indicator is more for website sections requiring payment to enter those areas or to access a set of premium services. Code as yes a subscription service that is available for a premium fee. Count as yes if the user has to pay a fixed annual subscription fee, even if, in addition, the user has to pay user fees. Most subscription services have a "home page" on the portal and provide services on various agency websites—code as yes for both the portal and the individual agency websites where the subscription services are found.

Site meets W3C disability guidelines: 0: no, 1: yes. To evaluate this, use the Bobby software on your computer. Choose the W3C guidelines by clicking Tools; Project Properties; Report Data; Accessibility; W3C Priority One Issues; OK. Scan the first page of each site by clicking Tools; Project Properties; What to Scan; Scan Limits; 1 page. Go back to the main page. Type in the URL for the front page of the website you are evaluating and click on submit to determine whether the site meets this set of guidelines. There will be a report indicating whether the site meets or does not meet the guidelines.

Has a privacy policy on site: 0: no, 1: yes. Code as yes if there is any mention of the privacy policy of the particular website, even if it merely says the site has a privacy policy. Sometimes, a privacy policy can be found at the bottom of the page under "About Us," "Privacy," or "Copyright." Occasionally the privacy policy only appears on the page where the user has to input information. Try searching Google for "site: www.site.gov privacy policy" or "site: www.site.gov privacy statement."

Privacy policy prohibits commercial marketing of user information: 0: no, 1: yes. The privacy policy states that it does not give, sell, or rent user information to third parties. Can also code as yes if the policy states that user information will only be used for the purpose for which it was submitted.

Site prohibits creation of permanent cookies or individual profiles of visitors: 0: no, 1: yes. Most privacy policies state whether they use *session cookies* (which are deleted when the browser is closed) or *permanent cookies* (which are saved on the hard drive) or both. Code as yes if the privacy policy prohibits permanent cookies and as no if it does not.

Site prohibits sharing personal information without prior consent of user: 0: no, 1: yes. The website will only share personal information (such as giving your home address) with your consent and to specifically answer your question. Passing information to law enforcement authorities would not be coded as yes since that is a noncommercial reason for sharing personal information.

Site can share personal information with legal authorities or law enforcement: 0: no, 1: yes. The website will share the user's personal information with legal authorities, law enforcement, or a court under a court order. Sometimes the policy specifically states that it will share with law enforcement if necessary, while other times the policy states that it will disclose "when permissible."

Has a visible security policy: 0: no, 1: yes. The security policy is its own distinct link or is part of the privacy policy. Once again, any mention of the policy is adequate for coding as yes. If the site is listed as being secure, that would be coded as having a visible security policy too.

Security policy uses computer software to monitor network traffic: 0: no, 1: yes. Almost all security policies with this feature will distinctly say that they use computer software to monitor network traffic. The website may not specifically say it uses software; it might say it tracks IP addresses, domains, browser types, and so on. Aesthetic or informational features such as web counters do not count.

Has official government services available to citizens: 0: no, 1: yes. This can take a variety of forms. Think of services as something that a citizen can conduct entirely on the website, without having to mail something in, make a phone call, or visit an office. Often, the transaction is an actual state service such as ordering a motor license, registering to vote, applying for a business permit, filing taxes online, ordering a publication, and filling out an online application and electronically submitting it directly to the department. Services must provide features where citizens and businesses apply for a service online and receive some tangible product or benefit in return. If one has to order a service online and then mail something in to execute the service, it cannot be considered as a fully online transaction and, therefore, the service is not considered an online service. Entering Social Security numbers to check tax refund status would be considered a service since one is not merely entering information but the government is providing specialized information to the user. Databases that generate customized results for the user count as services. Dynamic maps showing status of major highways count as services. Databases of judicial opinions, legislative bills, and attorney general opinions count as services. But mere text—whether on a web page or on an online publication—does not count. The transaction must involve inputting information, whether personal details or database queries. Furthermore, many websites have service links that provide no actual online services (instead they just provide information on different programs run by the agency), so it is important to check the links specifically for that purpose. Another important note is that even if the link to an online service connects the user to a different department to complete the transaction, it still counts as a service for that site. This is often seen on the state portal pages, as they document many of the services available on all of the different agencies' sites.

Has services requiring a user fee: 0: no, 1: yes. Fee is required to execute a particular service online. For example, if a driver's license costs $25 and the citizen has to pay $25 online, that would not be a user fee. It is just the normal fee for the service. If, however, the agency charges a $3 processing fee on top of the $25, that would be a user fee.

Number of different services: code actual number (0 if none). Simply count the number of online services. A site offering both hunting and fishing licenses would be coded as 2 for two services, since each serves different needs and different audiences.

Allows digital signatures on transactions: 0: no, 1: yes. Code as yes if the website specifically mentions that it has digital signature capabilities. Otherwise, code as no. (If not apparent, code as no as well.)

Allows payments using a credit card: 0: no, 1: yes. The website has the capability to use a credit card to complete the online transactions. Code as yes even if the link to use the credit card takes the user to an external site to enter the information. This often is found in conjunction with services or publications that can be ordered with a credit card. (If not apparent, code as no as well.)

Can e-mail department: 0: no, 1: yes. Any type of e-mail address for any person or division in the department is coded as yes. Even when there is not a specific e-mail address but there is a specific form that can be filled for comments, questions, or suggestions and submitted online it counts as yes. This type of situation is found on the websites of large agencies and top elected officials. The e-mail address of the webmaster does not count, but a general agency address (info@agency.gov) does, often located in the Contact Us section.

Has an area to post comments: 0: no, 1: yes. These take the form of user surveys, bulletin boards, chat rooms, or guest books. A comment form that generates an e-mail to the office counts (it also counts for the e-mail category above). Simply listing an address to e-mail comments and suggestions does not count.

Has an option for automatic e-mail updates, newsletters, or RSS and XML feeds: 0: no, 1: yes. The website gives the user the ability to sign up and register online to receive agency updates in such forms as newsletters, late-breaking news, and website notifications. These updates then are sent out to people who have registered to receive information or notifications.

Allows personalization of website: 0: no, 1: yes. This is a website where the user can customize it to the user's particular interests, often referred to as "MyNC." This can mean either customization for the individual user or customization based on various constituencies (for example, different pages specialized for parents, students, tourists, or teachers).

Has PDA or handheld access: 0: no, 1: yes. This would include access to the government website through a pager or mobile phone or access through any kind of personal digital assistant (as opposed to computer access through the Internet). Often, this capability is prominently mentioned on the homepage.

Flesch-Kincaid Grade Level Readability: Code the actual number. From the front page of the government website, copy the text by clicking Edit, Select All, and then Edit, Copy. Minimize this screen, and open a new blank Microsoft Word document. Click Edit and Paste to move this website text into the document. To set the computer to display readability statistics in Microsoft Word, click on Tools, Spelling and Grammar, Options, and check box for "Show readability statistics," and then click OK. To check the text pasted into the Word document, click on Tools and Spelling and Grammar (or the ABC icon on the ruler). Keep clicking on Ignore All until one comes to the end of the text when the readability statistics are displayed. The Flesch-Kincaid Grade Level Readability number is at the bottom of this display. Round to the closest whole number and enter this one- or two-digit number into the database. If the page generates a "0" score, open a new blank document and paste the contents of the website by going to Edit, Paste Special, and Unformatted Text. This still might not work: some sites imbed their text in an image file that Word cannot read.

Discloses site sponsorship: 0: no, 1: yes. This refers to whether the site indicates which organization is sponsoring the website.

Level of detail in the disclosure of site sponsorship: 1: a little, 2: some, 3: a lot of detail about the organization sponsoring the site. "A little" would be name, address, or phone number; "some" would refer to information regarding organization activities, and "a lot" would include material on what the organization has done, what its goals are, who contributes to the organization, and what its products are.

Type of site sponsorship: 1: for commercial or for profit, 2: for non-profit.

Number of illnesses or diseases discussed on the website (niche targeting): Code the actual number of illnesses or diseases that are dealt with on the site, up to 25 (anything more than 25 would be coded as 25).

Targets specific groups such as the poor, the elderly, the disabled, or people having particular diseases: 0: no, 1: yes.

Site information includes products, treatments, or drugs developed by the site sponsor: 0: no, 1: yes.

Has advertising from the site sponsor: 0: no, 1: yes.

Notes

CHAPTER ONE

1. The website address is www.hospitalcompare.hhs.gov. Kevin Freking, "Patients' Ratings of Hospitals Available Online," *Providence Journal,* March 29, 2008, p. A2.

2. Nancy Ferris, "Panelists' Consensus on E-Prescribing," *Government Health IT,* May 9, 2008.

3. Matthew Perrone, "Doctors Resist Electronic Prescriptions," *Providence Journal,* February 20, 2008, p. F2.

4. Helen Hughes Evans, "High Tech vs 'High Touch': The Impact of Medical Technology on Patient Care," in *Sociomedical Perspectives on Patient Care,* edited by Jeffrey M. Clair and Richard M. Allman (University Press of Kentucky, 1993), pp. 83–95.

5. Edward Alan Miller, "Telemedicine and Doctor-Patient Communication," *Journal of Telemedicine and Telecare* 7 (2001): 1–17. Also see Edward A. Miller, "The Technical and Interpersonal Aspects of Telemedicine: Effects on Doctor-Patient Communication," *Journal of Telemedicine and Telecare* 9 (2003): 1–7.

6. John Glaser, *The Strategic Application of Information Technology in Health Care Organizations* (San Francisco: Jossey-Bass, 2002).

7. Monica Murero and Ronald Rice, *The Internet and Health Care: Theory, Research, and Practice* (Mahway, N.J.: Lawrence Erlbaum Associates, 2006). For earlier treatments of this subject, see Ronald Rice and James Katz, *The Internet and Health Communication* (Thousand Oaks, Calif.: Sage, 2001), and Pam Whitten and David Cook, *Understanding Health Communications Technologies* (San Francisco: Jossey-Bass, 2004).

8. Jeff Goldsmith, *Digital Medicine: Implications for Healthcare Leaders* (Chicago: Health Administration Press, 2003).

9. PR Newswire, "Few Patients Use or Have Access to Online Services for Communicating with Their Doctors," September 22, 2006 (www.prnews wire.com [November 18, 2008]).

10. Ibid.

11. Susannah Fox, *Online Health Search 2006* (Washington: Pew Internet and American Life Project, October 29, 2006).

12. Gordon Brown, Tamara Stone, and Timothy Patrick, *Strategic Management of Information Systems in Healthcare* (Chicago: Health Administration Press, 2005).

13. Christine Borger and others, "Health Spending Projections through 2015," *Health Affairs* 25, no. 2 (2006): w61–w73; and Robert Pear, "Health Spending Exceeded Record $2 Trillion in 2006," *New York Times,* January 8, 2008, p. A20.

14. Ibid.

15. Pear, "Health Spending Exceeded Record $2 Trillion in 2006"; and Centers for Medicaid and Medicare Services, "Annual Report of the Boards of Trustees of the Federal Hospital Insurance and Federal Supplementary Medical Insurance Trust Funds" (2006).

16. Kaiser Family Foundation and Health Research and Educational Trust, *Employee Health Benefits: 2005 Annual Survey* (Washington: September 2005).

17. Judith A. Hall, Debra L. Roter, and N. R. Katz, "Meta-Analysis of Correlates Provider Behavior in Medical Encounters," *Medical Care* 26, no. 7 (1988): 657–75; Robert J. Blendon and others, "Health Care in the 2004 Presidential Election," *New England Journal of Medicine* 351, no. 13 (2004): 1314–22; and Barbara Starfield, "Is U.S. Health Really the Best in the World?" *Journal of the American Medical Association* 284, no. 4 (2000): 483–85.

18. Todd Gilmer and Richard Kronick, "It's the Premiums, Stupid: Projections of the Uninsured through 2013," *Health Affairs,* April 5, 2005 (http://content.healthaffairs.org/cgi/content/full/hlthaff.w5.143/DC1 [November 18, 2008]).

19. James Morone and Lawrence Jacobs, *Healthy, Wealthy, and Fair: Health Care and the Good Society* (Oxford University Press, 2005).

20. Robert J. Blendon and others, "Views of Practicing Physicians and the Public on Medical Errors," *New England Journal of Medicine* 347, no. 24 (2002): 1933–40; and Michelle M. Mello, Carly N. Kelly, and Troyen A. Brennan, "Fostering Rational Regulation of Patient Safety," *Journal of Health Politics, Policy, and Law* 30, no. 3 (2005): 375–426.

21. U.S. Newswire, "AARP, Business Roundtable, and SEIU Deliver Endorsed Health IT Principles to Congress," June 13, 2007 (www.newsunfiltered.com/archives/2007/06/aarp_business_r.html [November 18, 2008]).

22. Thomas H. Gallagher and others, "Patients' Attitudes toward Cost Control

Bonuses for Managed Care Physicians," *Health Affairs* 20, no. 2 (2001): 186–92; and Bruce E. Landon and others, "Health Plan Characteristics and Consumer Assessments of Quality," *Health Affairs* 20, no. 2 (2001): 274–86.

23. DataMonitor NewsWire, "Report Finds Healthcare IT Spending Increasing," July 13, 2006 (www.datamonitor.com/industries/news/article/?pid=93E7 F938-6482-42D1-88D7-40F8705A4D40&type=NewsWire [November 18, 2007]); and Darrell M. West, *Digital Government: Technology and Public Sector Innovation* (Princeton University Press, 2005).

24. Newt Gingrich with Dana Pavey and Anne Woodbury, *Saving Lives and Saving Money: Transforming Health and Healthcare* (Washington: Alexis de Tocqueville Institution, 2003).

25. HillaryClinton.com, "American Health Choices Plan," September 17, 2007 (www.hillaryclinton.com/news/speech/view/?id=3329 [November 18, 2008]). Also see Patrick Healy and Robin Toner, "Wary of Past, Clinton Unveils a Health Plan," *New York Times*, September 18, 2007, p. A1; and Perry Bacon Jr. and Anne Kornblut, "Clinton Presents Plan for Universal Coverage," *Washington Post*, September 18, 2007, p. A1.

26. BarackObama.com, "Barack Obama's Plan for a Healthy America" (www.barackobama.com/pdf/HealthPlanOverview.pdf [November 18, 2008]).

27. Richard Hillestad and others, "Can Electronic Medical Record Systems Transform Health Care? Potential Health Benefits, Savings, and Costs," *Health Affairs* 24, no. 5 (2005): 1103–17.

28. E. Andrew Balas and others, "Electronic Communication with Patients: Evaluation of Distance Medicine Technology," *Journal of the American Medical Association* 278, no. 2 (1997): 152–59.

29. Chen-Tan Lin and others, "An Internet-Based Patient-Provider Communication System: Randomized Controlled Trial," *Journal of Medical Internet Research* 7, no. 4 (2005): 47.

30. Jay J. Shen, "Health Information Technology: Will It Make Higher Quality and More Efficient Healthcare Delivery Possible?" *International Journal of Public Policy* 2, no. 3–4 (2007): 281–97.

31. Figures taken from John Glaser, testimony before Senate Committee on Veterans' Affairs, *Information Technology*, 110 Cong., September 19, 2007.

32. PR Newswire, "Few Patients Use or Have Access to Online Services for Communicating with their Doctors."

33. Christopher Sciamanna and others, "Unmet Needs of Primary Care Patients in Using the Internet for Health-Related Activities," *Journal of Medical Internet Research* 4, no. 3 (December 31, 2002): e19.

34. Darrell West, Diane Heith, and Chris Goodwin, "Harry and Louise Go to Washington," *Journal of Health Politics, Policy, and Law* 21, no. 1 (Spring 1996).

35. Gerard Anderson and others, "Health Care Spending and Use of Information Technology in OECD Countries," *Health Affairs* 25, no. 1 (2006): 819-31.

36. William G. Weissert and Edward A. Miller, "Punishing the Pioneers: The Medicare Modernization Act and State Pharmacy Assistance Programs," *Publius: The Journal of Federalism* 35, no. 1 (2005): 115–41.

37. Darrell West and Edward Alan Miller, "The Digital Divide in Public E-Health: Barriers to Accessibility and Privacy in State Health Department Websites," *Journal of Health Care for the Poor and Underserved* 17 (2006): 652–67.

38. Edward Alan Miller and Darrell West, "Where's the Revolution? Digital Technology and Health Care Communication in the Internet Age," forthcoming, *Journal of Health Politics, Policy, and Law* 34, no. 1 (March 2009); Ronald Rice, "Influences, Usage, and Outcomes of Internet Health Information Searching: Multivariate Results from the Pew Surveys," *International Journal of Medical Informatics* 75, no. 1 (2006): 8–28; Susannah Fox, "Prescription Drugs Online: One in Four Americans Have Looked Online for Drug Information, but Few Have Ventured into the Online Drug Marketplace" (Washington: PEW Internet and American Life Project, October 10, 2004); Susannah Fox, "Health Information Online: Eight in Ten Internet Users Have Looked for Health Information Online, with Increased Interest in Diet, Fitness, Drugs, Health Insurance, Experimental Treatments, and Particular Doctors and Hospitals"(Washington: Pew Internet and American Life Project, May 2005); Michelle L. Ybarra and Michael Suman, "Help-Seeking Behavior and the Internet: A National Survey," *International Journal of Medical Informatics* 75, no. 1 (January 2006): 29–41; Laurence Baker and others, "Use of the Internet and E-mail for Health Care Information," *Journal of the American Medical Association* 289, no. 18 (2003): 2400–06.

39. Betty L. Chang and others, "Bridging the Digital Divide: Reaching Vulnerable Populations," *Journal of the American Medical Informatics Association* 11, no. 6 (2004): 448–57.

40. David R. Williams, "Patterns and Causes of Disparities in Health," in *Policy Challenges in Modern Health Care,* edited by D. Mechanic and others (Rutgers University Press, 2005), pp. 115–34.

41. Susannah Fox, "Digital Divisions: There Are Clear Differences among Those with Broadband Connections, Dial-Up Connections, and No Connections at All to the Internet" (Washington: PEW Internet and American Life Project, October 5, 2005).

42. Miller and West, "Where's the Revolution?"; Rice, "Influences, Usage, and Outcomes of Internet Health Information Searching"; Fox, "Prescription Drugs Online"; Fox, "Health Information Online"; Ybarra and Suman, "Help-Seeking Behavior and the Internet"; Baker and others, "Use of the Internet and E-mail for Health Care Information."

43. Ahmad Risk and Carolyn Petersen, "Health Information on the Internet," *Journal of the American Medical Association* 287, no. 20 (2002): 2713–15; and Gunther Eysenbach and others, "Empirical Studies Assessing the Quality of Health Information for Consumers on the World Wide Web," *Journal of the American Medical Association* 287, no. 20 (2002): 2691–700.

44. Mark Kutner, E. Greenberg, and J. Baer, "A First Look at the Literacy of America's Adults in the 21st Century" (Washington: National Center for Education Statistics, December 2005).

45. Gloria Mayer and Michael Villaire, "Low Health Literacy and Its Effects on Patient Care," *Journal of Nursing Administration* 34, no. 10 (2004): 400–42; and Norah Shire, "Effects of Race, Ethnicity, Gender, Culture, Literacy, and Social Marketing on Public Health," *Journal of Gender Specific Medicine* 5, no. 2 (2002): 48–54.

46. Richard Wootton, Laurel S. Jebamani, and S. A. Dow, "E-Health and the Universitas 21 Organization, Telemedicine and Underserved Populations," *Journal of Telemedicine and Telecare* 11, no. 5 (2005): 221–24.

47. Michael Christopher, *E-Health Solutions for Healthcare Disparities* (New York: Springer, 2007).

48. DataMonitor NewsWire, "Report Finds Healthcare IT Spending Increasing."

49. Rainu Kaushal and others, "The Costs of a National Health Information Network," *Annals of American Medicine* 143, no. 3 (August 2, 2005): 165–73.

50. Gerard Anderson and others, "Health Care Spending and Use of Information Technology in OECD Countries," *Health Affairs* 25, no. 3 (2006): 819–31.

51. Ibid.

52. U.S. Department of Health and Human Services, "Health Information Technology Initiative Major Accomplishments: 2004–2006" (www.dhhs.gov/healthit/news/Accomplishments2006.html [January 26, 2009]).

53. Matthew DoBias, "EHR Adoption 'Pitifully Behind,'" *Modern Healthcare,* October 16, 2006, p. 8.

54. Eysenbach and others, "Empirical Studies Assessing the Quality of Health Information for Consumers on the World Wide Web"; and Edward Miller and Darrell West, "Where's the Revolution? Digital Technology and Health Care Communication in the Internet Age,"paper presented at the American Political Science Association Conference, August 31–September 3, 2006.

55. West, *Digital Government.*

56. Eysenbach and others, "Empirical Studies Assessing the Quality of Health Information for Consumers on the World Wide Web."

57. Fox, *Online Health Search 2006.*

58. David Shore, *The Trust Crisis in Healthcare: Causes, Consequences, and Cures* (Oxford University Press, 2007).

59. PR Newswire, "The Benefits of Electronic Medical Records Sound Good, but Privacy Could Become a Difficult Issue", February 8, 2007 (www.prnewswire.com/cgi-bin/stories.pl?ACCT=104&STORY=/www/story/02-08-2007/0004 523994&EDATE= [November 18, 2008]).

60. Ibid.

61. Janlori Goldman and Zoe Hudson, "Virtually Exposed: Privacy and E-Health," *Health Affairs* 19, no. 6 (November-December 2000). This article quoted from a January 2000 survey of Internet users conducted for the California Health Care Foundation entitled "Ethics Survey of Consumer Attitudes about Health Web Sites" (www.chcf.org/press/view.cfm?itemID=12277 [November 18, 2008]).

62. Marilyn Larkin, "New Reports Emphasize E-Health Privacy Concerns," *The Lancet* 357, no. 9274 (June 30, 2001): 2147.

63. Harris Poll, "Many U.S. Adults Are Satisfied with Use of Their Personal Health Information," March 26, 2007 (www.harrisinteractive.com/harris_poll/index.asp?PID=743 [November 18, 2008]).

64. James Anderson, "Social, Ethical, and Legal Barriers to E-Health," *International Journal of Medical Informatics* 76, no. 5–6 (May-June 2007): 480–83.

65. Ibid.

CHAPTER TWO

1. Nicholas Castle and Timothy Lowe, "Report Cards and Nursing Homes," *The Gerontologist* 45, no. 1 (February 2005): 48–67; Martin Marshall and others, "The Public Release of Performance Data: What Do We Expect to Gain? A Review of the Evidence," *Journal of the American Medical Association* 283, no. 14 (August 2005): 1866–74; and Mark Chassin, "Achieving and Sustaining Improved Quality: Lessons from New York State and Cardiac Surgery," *Health Affairs* 21, no. 4 (July-August 2002): 40–51.

2. Gunther Eysenbach, E. Sa, and T. Diepgen, "Shopping around the Internet Today and Tomorrow," *British Medical Journal* 319 (1999): 1294–98; and Maria Branni and James Anderson, "E-Medicine and Health Care Consumers," *Health Care Analysis* 10 (2002): 403–15.

3. Steve Lohr, "Dr. Google and Dr. Microsoft," *New York Times,* August 14, 2007, p. C1; and Milt Freudenheim, "AOL Founder Hopes to Build New Giant among a Bevy of Health Care Web Sites, *New York Times,* April 16, 2007, p. C1.

4. Edward Clark, "Health Care Web Sites: Are They Reliable?" *Journal of Medical Systems* 26, no. 6 (December 2002): 519–28.

5. Maria Branni and James Anderson, "E-Medicine and Health Care Consumers," *Health Care Analysis* 10 (2002): 403–15.

6. "For Drug Makers, Full Disclosure on the Web Can Pose Problems," *Providence Journal*, May 23, 2007, p. A4.

7. Clark, "Health Care Web Sites."

8. Mary Anne Bright and others, "Exploring E-Health Usage and Interest among Cancer Information Service Users," *Journal of Health Communication* 10 (2005): 35–52.

9. Rowena Cullen, *Health Information on the Internet: A Study of Providers, Quality, and Users* (Westport, Conn.: Praeger, 2006).

10. Clark, "Health Care Web Sites."

11. Gretchen Berland and others, "Health Information on the Internet: Accessibility, Quality, and Readability in English and Spanish," *Journal of the American Medical Association* 285 (May 23, 2001): 2612–21.

12. Branni and Anderson, "E-Medicine and Health Care Consumers."

13. Ahmad Risk and Carolyn Petersen, "Health Information on the Internet," *Journal of the American Medical Association* 287, no. 20 (2002): 2713–15.

14. Judith Waldrop and Sharon Stern, *Disability Status* (U.S. Census Bureau, 2003).

15. "Language, School Enrollment, and Educational Attainment," U.S. Census Bureau, 2000 (http://factfinder.census.gov).

16. John Miller, "English Is Broken Here," *Policy Review* (September-October 1996).

17. Irwin Kirsch and others, *Adult Literacy in America* (Washington: National Center for Education Statistics, 1993).

18. Carl Kaestle, "Formal Education and Adult Literacy Proficiencies: Exploring the Relevance of Gender, Race, Age, Income, and Parents' Education," *Adult Literacy and Education in America* (U.S. Department of Education, 2001).

19. David Howard, Julie Gazmararian, and Ruth Parker, "The Impact of Low Health Literacy on the Medical Costs of Medicare Managed Care Enrollees," *American Journal of Medicine* 118, no. 4 (April 2005): 371–77; J. Gazmararian and others, "Public Health Literacy in America: An Ethical Perspective," *American Journal of Preventive Medicine* 28, no. 3 (April 2005): 317–22; and Dean Schillinger and others, "Association of Health Literacy with Diabetes Outcomes," *Journal of the American Medical Association* 288, no. 4 (July 2002): 475–82.

20. Scott Ratzen and Ruth Parker, "Introduction," in *National Library of Medicine Current Bibliographies in Medicine: Health Literacy*, edited by C. Selden and others (Bethesda, Md.: National Institutes of Health, 2000).

21. Council on Scientific Affairs, "Health Literacy," *Journal of the American Medical Association* 281, no. 6 (February 10, 1999): 552–57.

22. Norah Shire, "Effects of Race, Ethnicity, Gender, Culture, Literacy, and Social Marketing on Public Health," *Journal of Gender Specific Medicine* 5, no.

2 (March-April 2002): 48–54; Charles Bennett and others, "Relation between Literacy, Race, and Stage of Presentation among Low-Income Patients with Prostate Cancer," *Journal of Clinical Oncology* 16 (1998): 3101–04; and Michael Paasche-Orlow and others, "The Prevalence of Limited Health Literacy," *Journal of General Internal Medicine* 20 (2005): 175–84.

23. Gloria Mayer and Michael Villaire, "Low Health Literacy and Its Effects on Patient Care," *Journal of Nursing Administration* 34, no. 10 (October 2004): 440–42.

24. Rudolph Flesch, *Flesch-Kincaid Readability Formula* (Boston: Houghton-Mifflin, 1965).

25. Council for Excellence in Government, "The New E-Government Equation," April 2003 ((www.excelgov.org).

26. Ibid.

27. Janlori Goldman and Zoe Hudson, "Virtually Exposed: Privacy and E-Health," *Health Affairs* 19, no. 6 (November-December 2000): 140–48.

28. David Wahlberg, "Patient Records Exposed on Web," *Ann Arbor News*, February 10, 1999, p.1.

29. Goldman and Hudson, "Virtually Exposed."

30. Marilyn Larkin, "New Reports Emphasize E-Health Privacy Concerns," *The Lancet* 357, no. 9274 (June 30, 2001): 2147.

31. Alejandro R. Jadad and Anna Gagliardi, "Rating Health Information on the Internet: Navigating to Knowledge or to Babel?" *Journal of the American Medical Association* 279, no. 8 (1998): 611–14; and Gretchen P. Purcell, P. Wilson, and T. Delamothe, "The Quality of Information on the Internet," *British Medical Journal* 324 (2002): 557–58.

32. Gunther Eysenbach and others, "Empirical Studies Assessing the Quality of Health Information for Consumers on the World Wide Web," *Journal of the American Medical Association* 287, no. 20 (2002): 2691–700.

33. Clark, "Health Care Web Sites."

34. Ben Shneiderman, "Universal Usability," *Communications of the ACM* 43 (2000): 85–91.

35. Martin Gould, "Switzer Seminar Series Remarks," Michigan State University, October 4, 2001.

36. David Blumenthal, "Doctors in a Wired World: Can Professionalism Survive Connectivity?" *Milbank Quarterly* 80, no. 3 (2002): 525–46.

CHAPTER THREE

1. Jeannette Borzo, "A New Physician's Assistant," *Wall Street Journal*, October 10, 2005, p. R5.

2. Anne Marie Audet and others, "Information Technologies: When Will They Make It into Physicians' Black Bags?" *Medscape General Medicine* 6, no. 4 (2004): 2.

3. James G. Anderson and E. Andrew Balas, "Computerization of Primary Care in the U.S.," *International Journal of Health Information Systems and Informatics* 1, no. 3 (2006): 1–23. Also see James G. Anderson and E. A. Balas, "Information Technology in Primary Care Practice in the United States," in *Healthcare Information Systems and Informatics,* edited by Joseph Tan (Hershey, Pa.: Information Science Publishing, 2008); Catherine Burt, E. Hing, and D. Woodwell, "Electronic Medical Record Use by Office-Based Physicians," unpublished paper, Centers for Disease Control and Prevention, 2005; and Ashish Jha and others, "How Common Are Electronic Health Records in the United States?" *Health Affairs* 25, no. 5 (2006): p. 2496-w507.

4. Darrell M. West, *The Rise and Fall of the Media Establishment* (Boston: Bedford/St. Martin's Press, 2001), p. 59.

5. Mary Anne Bright and others, "Exploring E-Health Usage and Interest among Cancer Information Service Users," *Journal of Health Communication* 10 (2005): 35–52.

6. Ronald Andersen, "Revisiting the Behavior Model and Access to Care: Does It Matter?" *Journal of Health and Social Behavior* 36, no. 1 (1995): 1–10; and Ronald Andersen and J. Newman, "Societal and Individual Determinants of Medical Care Utilization in the United States,"*Milbank Memorial Fund Quarterly* 51 (Winter 1973): 95–124.

7. Karen B. DeSalvo and others, "Mortality Prediction with a Single General Self-Rated Health Question: A Meta-Analysis," *Journal of General Internal Medicine* 21, no. 3 (2006): 267–75; and Ingeborg Eriksson, A. L. Unden, and S. Elofsson, "Self-Rated Health: Comparisons between Three Different Measures,"*International Journal of Epidemiology* 30, no. 2: 326–33.

8. Catherine R. Selden and others, *Health Literacy: January 1990 through October 1999,* Current Bibliographies in Medicine 2000-1 (Bethesda, Md.: National Library of Medicine, February 2000).

9. Lisa D. Chew, K. A. Bradley, and E. J. Boyko, "Brief Questions to Identify Patients with Inadequate Health Literacy," *Family Medicine* 36, no. 8 (2004): 588–94.

10. Grant Marshall and Ron Hays, *The Patient Satisfaction Questionnaire Short Form (PSQ-18)* (Santa Monica, Calif.: RAND, 1994).

11. Laurence Baker and others, "Use of the Internet and E-Mail for Health Care Information," *Journal of the American Medical Association* 289, no. 18 (2003): 2400–06.

12. James Katz and Ronald Rice, *Social Consequences of Internet Use* (MIT Press, 2002). Also see Barry Wellman and Caroline Haythornthwaite, *The Internet in Everyday Life* (Oxford: Blackwell Publishers, 2002).

13. Margaret Lethbridge-Cejku, D. Rose, and J. Vickerie, "Summary Health Statistics for U.S. Adults: National Health Interview Survey 2004," *Vital and Health Statistics,* series 10, no. 228 (Hyattsville, Md.: National Centers for Health Statistics, 2006).

14. Susannah Fox, "Health Information Online: Eight in Ten Internet Users Have Looked for Health Information Online, with Increased Interest in Diet, Fitness, Drugs, Health Insurance, Experimental Treatments, and Particular Doctors and Hospitals" (Washington: Pew Internet and American Life Project, May 2005); Ronald E. Rice, "Influences, Usage, and Outcomes of Internet Health Information Searching: Multivariate Results from the Pew Surveys," *International Journal of Medical Informatics* 75, no. 1 (2006): 8–28; Mollyanne Brodie and others, "Health Information, the Internet, and the Digital Divide," *Health Affairs* 19, no. 6 (2000): 255–65; Michelle L. Ybarra and Michael Suman, "Help-Seeking Behavior and the Internet: A National Survey," *International Journal of Medical Informatics* 75, no. 1 (January 2006), pp. 29–41.

15. Suzanne Dickerson and others, "Patient Internet Use for Health Information at Three Urban Primary Care Clinics," *Journal of the American Medical Informatics Association* 11, no. 6 (2004): 499–504.

16. Susannah Fox, "Prescription Drugs Online: One in Four Americans Has Looked Online for Drug Information, but Few Have Ventured Into the Online Drug Marketplace" (Washington: PEW Internet and American Life Project, October 10, 2004); Baker and others, "Use of the Internet and E-Mail for Health Care Information."

17. Susannah Fox and D. Fallows, "Internet Health Resources: Health Searches and E-Mail have Become Commonplace, but There is Room for Improvement in Searches and Overall Internet Access" (Washington: Pew Internet and American Life Project, July 16, 2003).

18. Dawn Misra, "Women's Health Data Book. A Profile of Women's Health in the United States," 3rd ed. (Washington: Jacobs Institute of Women's Health and the Henry J. Kaiser Family Foundation, 2001).

19. Lethbridge-Cejku, Rose, and Vickerie, "Summary Health Statistics for U.S. Adults: National Health Interview Survey 2004"; Rice, "Influences, Usage, and Outcomes of Internet Health Information Searching: Multivariate Results form the Pew Surveys"; Ybarra and Suman, "Help-Seeking Behavior and the Internet: A National Survey."

20. Kelvin Jordan, B. N. Ong, and P. Croft, "Previous Consultation and Self-Reported Health Status as Predictors of Future Demand for Primary Care," *Journal of Epidemiology and Community Health* 57, no. 2 (2003): 109–13; Rice, "Influences, Usage, and Outcomes of Internet Health Information Searching: Multivariate Results form the Pew Surveys"; Baker and others, "Use of the Internet and E-Mail for Health Care Information."

21. Joseph A. Diaz and others, "Patients' Use of the Internet for Medical Information," *Journal of General Internal Medicine* 17, no. 3 (2002): 180–85; Ybarra and Suman, "Help-Seeking Behavior and the Internet"; and Lethbridge-Cejku, Rose, and Vickerie, "Summary Health Statistics for U.S. Adults: National Health Interview Survey 2004."

22. Diaz and others, "Patients' Use of the Internet for Medical Information"; and Ybarra and Suman, "Help-Seeking Behavior and the Internet."

23. Edward Alan Miller, Darrell M. West, and Melanie Wasserman, "Health Information Websites: Characteristics of Users by Race and Ethnicity," *Journal of Telemedicine and Telecare* 13, no. 3 (September 2007): 298–302.

24. John Horrigan and K. Murray, "Rural Broadband Internet Use" (Washington: Pew Internet and American Life Project, February 2006).

25. Edward A. Miller, "Solving the Disjuncture between Research and Practice: Telehealth Trends in the 21st Century," *Health Policy* 82, no. 2 (July 2007): 133–141.

26. Bill Grigsby, *TRC Report on U.S. Telemedicine Activity with an Overview of Non-US Activity* (Kingston, N.J.: Civic Research Institute, 2004); Blackford Middleton, "Achieving U.S. Health Information Technology Adoption: The Need for a Third Hand," *Health Affairs* 24, no. 5 (2005): 1269–72.

27. Eugenie M. Komives, "Clinician-Patient E-Mail Communication Challenges for Reimbursement," *North Carolina Medical Journal* 66, no. 3 (2005): 238–40; Jonathan Rutland, C. Marie, and B. Rutland, "A System of Telephone and Secure E-Mail Consultations, with Automatic Billing," *Journal of Telemedicine and Telecare* 10, supp. 1 (2004): S1:88–S1:91.

28. Robert H. Miller and Ida Sim, "Physicians' Use of Electronic Medical Records," *Health Affairs* 23, no. 2 (2004): 116–26.

29. J. D. Kleinke, "Dot-gov: Market Failure and the Creation of a National Health Information Technology System," *Health Affairs* 24, no. 5 (2005): 1246–62.

CHAPTER FOUR

1. Laurence Baker and others, "Use of the Internet and E-Mail for Health Care Information," *Journal of the American Medical Association* 289, no. 18 (2003): 2400–06.

2. David Blumenthal, "Doctors in a Wired World: Can Professionalism Survive Connectivity?" *The Milbank Quarterly* 80, no. 3 (2002): 525–46.

3. Newt Gingrich with Dana Pavey and Anne Woodbury, *Saving Lives and Saving Money: Transforming Health and Healthcare* (Washington: Alexis de Tocqueville Institution, 2003).

4. Patrick Healy and Robin Toner, "Wary of Past, Clinton Unveils A Health Plan," *New York Times,* September 18, 2007, p. A1.

5. Richard Baron and others, "Electronic Health Records: Just around the Corner? Or over the Cliff?" *Annals of Internal Medicine* 143, no. 3 (August 2, 2005): 222–26.

6. Baker and others, "Use of the Internet and E-Mail for Health Care Information."

7. Karen Mossberger, Caroline Tolbert, and Mary Stansbury, *Virtual Inequality: Beyond the Digital Divide* (Georgetown University Press, 2003).

8. Blumenthal, "Doctors in a Wired World."

9. Mossberger, Tolbert, and Stansbury, *Virtual Inequality.*

10. Joseph A. Diaz and others, "Patients' Use of the Internet for Medical Information," *Journal of General Internal Medicine* 17, no. 3 (2002): 180–85.

11. Vicki Fung and others, "Early Experiences with E-Health Services," *Medical Care* 44, no. 5 (May 2006): 491–96.

12. Ronald Rice, "Influences, Usage, and Outcomes of Internet Health Information Searching: Multivariate Results from the Pew Surveys," *International Journal of Medical Informatics* 75, no. 1 (2006): 8–28.

CHAPTER FIVE

1. Michael Christopher Gibbons, *E-Health Solutions for Healthcare Disparities* (New York: Springer, 2007).

2. Mollyanne Brodie and others, "Health Information, the Internet, and the Digital Divide," *Health Affairs* 19, no. 6 (2000): 255–65.

3. *National Vital Statistics Reports* 52, no. 14 (February 18, 2004), p. 33, table 12.

4. Kevin Sack, "Research Finds Wide Disparities in Health Care by Race and Region," *New York Times,* June 5, 2008, p. A18.

5. Michael Millenson, "Want Universal Health Care? The Operative Word is 'Care,'" *Washington Post,* June 8, 2008, p B3.

6. Brodie and others, "Health Information, the Internet, and the Digital Divide"; and Ronald E. Rice, "Influences, Usage, and Outcomes of Internet Health Information Searching: Multivariate Results from the Pew Surveys," *International Journal of Medical Informatics* 75, no. 1 (2006): 8–28.

7. Suzanne Dickerson and others, "Patient Internet Use for Health Information at Three Urban Primary Care Clinics," *Journal of the American Medical Informatics Association* 11, no. 6 (2004): 499–504; and J. Hsu and others, "Use of E-Health Services between 1999 and 2002: A Growing Digital Divide," *Journal of the American Medical Informatics Association* 12 (2005): 164–71.

8. Michelle L. Ybarra and Michael Suman, "Help-Seeking Behavior and the

Internet: A National Survey," *International Journal of Medical Informatics* 75, no. 1 (January 2006): 29–41; and Lisa D. Chew, Katherine A. Bradley, and Edward J. Boyko, "Brief Questions to Identify Patients with Inadequate Health Literacy," *Family Medicine* 36 (2004): 588–94.

9. Susannah Fox, "Health Information Online: Eight in Ten Internet Users Have Looked for Health Information" (Washington: Pew Internet and American Life Project, May 2005).

10. Rice, "Influences, Usage, and Outcomes of Internet Health Information Searching."

11. Anne Case and Christina Paxson, "Children's Health and Social Mobility," *Future of Children* 16, no. 2 (Autumn 2006): 151–73.

12. Susannah Fox, "Digital Divisions" (Washington: PEW Internet and American Life Project, October 2005).

13. U.S. Department of Commerce, *A Nation Online: Entering the Broadband Age* (September 2006).

14. David R. Williams, *Patterns and Causes of Disparities in Health: Policy Challenges in Modern Health Care,* edited by D. Mechanic and others (Rutgers University Press, 2005), pp. 115–34.

15. Institute of Medicine, *Unequal Treatment: Confronting Racial and Ethnic Disparities in Health Care* (Washington: National Academy of Sciences, 2002).

16. James Katz and Ronald Rice, *Social Consequences of Internet Use* (MIT Press, 2002).

17. Karen Mossberger, Caroline Tolbert, and Mary Stansbury, *Virtual Inequality* (Georgetown University Press, 2003).

18. Mark Kutner, Elizabeth Greenberg, and Justin Baer, *A First Look at the Literacy of America's Adults in the 21st Century,* NCES 2006-470 (Washington: National Center for Education Statistics, U.S. Department of Education, December 2005).

19. U.S. Bureau of the Census, *2005 American Community Survey: B03002. Hispanic or Latino Origin by Race* (2006).

20. Mossberger, Tolbert, and Stansbury, *Virtual Inequality.*

21. Ibid.

22. Karen B. DeSalvo, "Mortality Prediction with a Single General Self-Rated Health Question," *Journal of General Internal Medicine* 21 (2006): 267–75.

23. Chew, Bradley, and Boyko, "Brief Questions to Identify Patients with Inadequate Health Literacy"; Brodie and others, "Health Information, the Internet, and the Digital Divide"; Rice, "Influences, Usage, and Outcomes of Internet Health Information Searching"; and Ybarra and Suman, "Help-Seeking Behavior and the Internet."

24. Brodie and others, "Health Information, the Internet, and the Digital Divide."

25. Fabio Sabogal, Joseph Scherger, and Ida Ahmadpour, "Supporting Care Management, Improving Care Coordination: The Role of Electronic Health Records," *California Association for Healthcare Quality* 32, no. 3 (2007).

26. Nilda Chong, *The Latino Patient: A Cultural Guide for Health Care Providers* (Yarmouth, Me.: Intercultural Press, 2002).

27. Kevin Sack, "Research Finds Wide Disparities in Health Care by Race and Region," *New York Times,* June 5, 2008, p. A18.

28. Dickerson and others, "Patient Internet Use for Health Information at Three Urban Primary Care Clinics"; and Ybarra and Suman, "Help-Seeking Behavior and the Internet."

29. Basmat Parsad and Jennifer Jones, "Internet Access in U.S. Public Schools and Classrooms: 1994–2003," NCES 2005-015 (Washington: National Center for Education Statistics, U.S. Department of Education, 2005).

30. Darrell M. West and Edward Alan Miller, "The Digital Divide in Public E-Health: Barriers to Accessibility and Privacy in State Health Department Websites," *Journal of Health Care for the Poor and Underserved* 17 (2006): 652–67.

31. Gunther Eysenbach and others,"Empirical Studies Assessing the Quality of Health Information for Consumers on the World Wide Web," *Journal of the American Medical Association* 287, no. 20 (2002): 2691–700.

32. "Health Literacy: A Report of the Council on Scientific Affairs," *Journal of the American Medical Association* 281 (1999): 552–57.

33. Josephine Marcotty, "A Health Makeover for an Entire Town," Scripps Howard News Service, June 12, 2008.

34. Ybarra and Suman, "Help-Seeking Behavior and the Internet."

35. National Center for Health Statistics, "Health, United States, 2005" (Hyattsville, Md.: 2005); U.S. Bureau of the Census, "Educational Attainment in the United States: 2004" (2006); and U.S. Bureau of the Census, "Age by Ethnicity by English Ability: Census 2000 Public Use Microsample (5% Sample)" (2006).

36. U.S. Bureau of the Census, "Educational Attainment in the United States: 2004."

CHAPTER SIX

1. Darrell M. West and Edward Alan Miller, "The Digital Divide in Public E-Health: Barriers to Accessibility and Privacy in State Health Department Websites," *Journal of Health Care for the Poor and Underserved* 17 (2006): 652–67.

2. Susannah Fox, "Health Information Online: Eight in Ten Internet Users Have Looked for Health Information Online, with Increased Interest in Diet, Fitness, Drugs, Health Insurance, Experimental Treatments, and Particular Doctors and Hospitals" (Washington: Pew Internet and American Life Project, May 2005); and Laurence Baker and others, "Use of the Internet and E-Mail for

Health Care Information," *Journal of the American Medical Association* 289, no. 18 (2003): 2400–06.

3. Edward Alan Miller, Darrell M.West, and Melanie Wasserman, "Health Information Websites: Characteristics of U.S. Users by Race and Ethnicity," *Journal of Telemedicine and Telecare* 13, no. 3 (September 2007): 298–302.

4. Mollyanne Brodie and others, "Health Information, the Internet, and the Digital Divide," *Health Affairs* 19, no. 6 (2000): 255–65; Ronald E. Rice, "Influences, Usage, and Outcomes of Internet Health Information Searching: Multivariate Results from the Pew Surveys," *International Journal of Medical Informatics* 75, no. 1 (2006): 8–28; Michelle L. Ybarra and Michael Suman, "Help-Seeking Behavior and the Internet: A National Survey," *International Journal of Medical Informatics* 75, no. 1 (January 2006): 29–41.

5. Baker and others, "Use of the Internet and E-mail for Health Care Information"; Brodie and others, "Health Information, the Internet, and the Digital Divide": and Betty L. Chang and others, "Bridging the Digital Divide: Reaching Vulnerable Populations," *Journal of the American Medical Informatics Association* 11, no. 6 (2004): 448–57.

6. Ybarra and Suman, "Help-Seeking Behavior and the Internet."

7. Chang and others, "Bridging the Digital Divide: Reaching Vulnerable Populations."

8. Ahmad Risk and Carolyn Petersen, "Health Information on the Internet," *Journal of the American Medical Association* 287, no. 20 (2002): 2713–715; and John Horrigan and K. Murray, "Rural Broadband Internet Use" (Washington: Pew Internet and American Life Project, February 2006).

9. Gunther Eysenbach and others, "Empirical Studies Assessing the Quality of Health Information for Consumers on the World Wide Web," *Journal of the American Medical Association* 287, no. 20 (2002): 2691–700; Alejandro Jadad and Anna Gagliardi, "Rating Health Information on the Internet: Navigating to Knowledge or to Babel?" *Journal of the American Medical Association* 279, no. 8 (1998): 611–14; and Gretchen P. Purcell, Petra Wilson, and Tony Delamothe, "The Quality of Information on the Internet," *British Medical Journal* 324, no. 7337 (2002): 557–58.

10. Darrell M. West, *Digital Government: Technology and Public Sector Performance* (Princeton University Press, 2005).

11. Shailagh Murray and Charles Babington, "New Offensive on Medicare Drug Benefit," *Washington Post,* February 28, 2006, p. A13.

12. Susannah Fox, "Wired Seniors: A Fervent Few, Inspired by Family Ties" (Washington: Pew Internet and American Life Project, September 2001).

13. Ibid.

14. Paul Abramson, John Aldrich, and David Rohde, *Change and Continuity in the 2004 Elections* (Washington: CQ Press, 2006).

15. West and Miller, "The Digital Divide in Public E-Health."

16. Mark Schlesinger and Bradford H. Gray, "How Nonprofits Matter in American Medicine and What to Do about It," *Health Affairs*, June 20, 2006 (http://content.healthaffairs.org/cgi/content/abstract/25/4/W287 [January 6, 2009]).

CHAPTER SEVEN

1. James Anderson, "Social, Ethical, and Legal Barriers to E-Health," *International Journal of Medical Informatics* 76, nos. 5–6 (May-June 2007): 480–83; and Bob Brewin, "The U.S. Health Care Community Is Not Alone in Its Struggles with Privacy," *Government Health*, September 2, 2005.

2. Monica Murero and Ronald Rice, *The Internet and Health Care: Theory, Research, and Practice* (Mahway, N.J.: Lawrence Erlbaum Associates, 2006). For earlier treatments of this subject, see Ronald Rice and James Katz, *The Internet and Health Communication* (Thousand Oaks, Calif.: Sage, 2001).

3. Darrell M. West, "Improving Technology Utilization in Electronic Government around the World: 2008," unpublished paper, Brookings, August 2008.

4. Hege K. Andreassen and others, "European Citizens' Use of E-Health Services: A Study of Seven Countries," *BMC Public Health* 7, no. 53 (2007).

5. Anderson, "Social, Ethical, and Legal Barriers to E-Health."

6. Cathy Schoen and others, "Toward Higher-Performance Health Systems," *Health Affairs* 26, no. 6 (November 1, 2007): w717–w734.

7. World Health Organization, "E-Health Resolution," 58th World Health Assembly, Geneva, May 25, 2005.

8. See "Global Observatory for E-Health" (www.who.int/kms/initiatives/ehealth/en [January 9, 2009]).

9. Jai Mohan and A. B. Suleiman, "E-Health Strategies for Developing Nations," in *Yearbook of Medical Informatics,* edited by R. Haux and C. Kulikowski (Stuttgart, Germany: Schattauer Verlagsgesellschaft, 2005), pp. 148–56. Also see Nancy Lorenzi, "E-Health Strategies Worldwide," in *Yearbook of Medical Informatics,* edited by Haux and Kulikowski, pp. 157–66.

10. Antoine Geissbuhler, R. Haux, and S. Kwankam, "Towards Health for All: WHO and IMIA Intensify Collaboration," *Methods of Informatics Medicine* 46, no. 5 (2007): 503–05.

11. Eurobarometer report can be found at http://ec.europa.eu/public_opinion/index_en.htm.

12. Anderson, "Social, Ethical, and Legal Barriers to E-Health."

13. Brewin, "The U.S. Health Care Community Is Not Alone in Its Struggles with Privacy."

14. D. Jane Bower and others, "Designing and Implementing E-Health Applications in the UK's National Health Service," *Journal of Health Communication* 10, no. 8 (December 2005): 733–50.

15. Roxana Dumitru and H. Prokosch, "German Healthcare Consumers' Use and Perception of the Internet and Related Technologies to Communicate with Healthcare Professionals," Lehrstuhl für Medizinische Informatik, Friedrich-Alexander Universität Erlangen-Nürnberg, *AMIA Annual Symposium Proceedings Archive* (2006), pp. 224–28.

16. The report can be found online at www.hineurope.com/Content/Default.asp?

17. Anderson, "Social, Ethical, and Legal Barriers to E-Health."

18. Rory Watson, "EU Wants Every Member to Develop a 'Roadmap' for E-Health," *BMJ* 328 (May 15, 2004): 1155.

19. Canada Newsire, "The Calgary Health Region Selects CGI to Advance E-Health Services," May 14, 2007.

20. Stephen Llewellyn, "Health Minister Envisions One Patient, One Record System," *Daily Gleaner,* May 18, 2007, p. A4.

21. Steven Mizrach, "Natives on the Electronic Frontier," Ph.D. dissertation, University of Florida, 1999.

22. Roberto Rocha, "Comforts of Home in Hospital," *Montreal Gazette,* November 21, 2006, p. B4.

23. Ibid.

24. Ian Holliday and Wai-keung Tam, "E-Health in the East Asian Tigers," *International Journal of Medical Informatics* 73, nos. 11–12 (November 2004): 759–69.

25. JCN Newswire, "Fujitsu Primequest Server Deployed for Integrated Hospital Information System at Nagoya University Hospital," March 9, 2007.

26. AFX News, "Australia's IBA to Put Up National Health Channel on China's BesTV Network," February 13, 2007.

27. This international initiative is summarized in "The INFO Project" (www.popline.org/docs/168413 [January 9, 2009]).

28. Eleanor Limprecht, "GPs Are Doing It for Themselves When It Comes to Shared Electronic Health Records," *Australian Doctor,* February 9, 2007.

29. "Onward and Upward," *Pharmacy News,* February 2007.

30. Brewin, "The U.S. Health Care Community Is Not Alone in Its Struggles with Privacy."

31. ACN Newswire, "IBA Health and Healthe Sign LOI for Health Records across SE Asia," May 1, 2007.

32. Brynn Wainstein and others, "Use of the Internet by Parents of Paediatric Patients," *Journal of Paediatrics and Child Health* 42 (2006): 528–32.

33. Ibid.

34. James Riley, "Data Privacy Key Consumer Concern," IT Security Expo Australia, August 30, 2007.

35. Joses Kirigia and others, "E-Health: Determinants, Opportunities, Challenges, and the Way forward for Countries in the WHO Africa Region," *BMC Public Health* 5 (December 20, 2005): 137–48.

36. Ibid.

37. Data come from the World Bank's Development Data Group (DECDG) databases (www.worldbank.org).

38. Data come from the World Bank's Development Data Group (DECDG) databases (www.worldbank.org). The political variables came from a shared global data set put together by Pippa Norris of Harvard University. Vanhanen's measure of political competition is described in Tatu Vanhanen, "A New Dataset for Measuring Democracy, 1810–1998," *Journal of Peace Research* 37, no. 2 (2000): 251–65.

CHAPTER EIGHT

1. Klaus Kuhn and others, "From Health Information Systems to E-Health," *Methods in Informatics Medicine* 46, no. 4 (2007): 450.

2. Klaus Kuhn and others, "Expanding the Scope of Health Information Systems," in *Yearbook of Medical Informatics,* edited by Reinhold Haux and C. Kulikowski (Stuttgart, Germany: Schattauer Verlagsgesellschaft, 2006), pp. 43–52.

3. Darrell M. West, *Digital Government: Technology and Public Sector Performance* (Princeton University Press, 2005).

4. John Horrigan, "A Typology of Information and Communication Technology Users" (Washington: Pew Internet and American Life Project, May 7, 2007).

5. Internet World Stats (www.InternetWorldStats.com [January 13, 2009]).

6. John Hsu and others, "Use of E-Health Services between 1999 and 2002: A Growing Digital Divide," *Journal of the American Medical Informatics Association* 12, no. 2 (March-April 2005): 164–71.

7. Ben Veenhof, Yvan Clermont, and George Sciadas, *Literacy and Digital Technologies* (Ottawa, Canada: Statistics Canada, 2005).

8. Institute of Medicine, *Health Literacy: A Prescription to End Confusion* (Washington: National Academies Press, 2004).

9. Cameron Norman and Harvey Skinner, "E-Health Literacy: Essential Skills for Consumer Health in a Networked World," *Journal of Medical Internet Research* 8, no. 2 (April-June 2006): e-9.

10. June Forkner-Dunn, "Internet-Based Patient Self-Care: The Next Generation of Health Care Delivery," *Journal of Medical Internet Research* 5, no. 2 (April-June 2003): e-8.

11. Tom Spooner, Lee Rainie, and Peter Meredith, "Asian Americans and the Internet" (Washington: Pew Internet and American Life Project, December 12, 2001); and Forkner-Dunn, "Internet-Based Patient Self-Care."

12. Pew Internet and American Life Project, "Tracking Online Life: How Women Use the Internet to Cultivate Relationships with Family and Friends"

(Washington: May 10, 2000); and John Powell and Aileen Clarke, "The WWW of the World Wide Web: Who, What, and Why?" *Journal of Medical Internet Research* 4, no. 1 (January-March 2002): e-4.

13. Nadine Wathen and Roma Harris, "How Rural Women Search for Health Information," *Qualitative Health Research* 17, no. 5 (May 2007): 639–51.

14. Joseph Wen and Joseph Tan, "The Evolving Face of TeleMedicine and E-Health," proceedings of the Thirty-Sixth Hawaii International Conference on System Sciences, January 6–9, 2003; and Steven O'Dell, "Realizing Positive Returns from Your E-Health Investment," *Healthcare Financial Management* 55, no. 2 (2001): 50–55.

15. Horrigan, "A Typology of Information and Communication Technology Users."

16. James Anderson, "Consumers of E-Health: Patterns of Use and Barriers," *Social Science Computer Review* 22 (2004): 242–48.

17. Harvey Skinner, Sherry Biscope, and Blake Poland, "Quality of Internet Access: Barrier behind Internet Use Statistics," *Social Science and Medicine* 57 (2003): 875–80.

18. Deborah Bowen and others, "Predictors of Women's Internet Access and Internet Health Seeking," *Health Care for Women International* 24, no. 10 (December 2003): 940–51.

19. Jim Finkle, "Nonprofit May Launch $350 Laptop by Christmas," *Boston Globe,* July 23, 2007.

20. Steve Lohr, "Buy a Laptop for a Child, Get Another Laptop Free," *New York Times,* September 24, 2007, p. C1.

21. Ibid.

22. World Bank, "World Development Indicators" (Washington: 2006).

23. Steve Goldberg and Nilmini Wickramasinghe, "21st Century Healthcare: The Wireless Panacea," proceedings of the Thirty-Sixth Hawaii International Conference on System Sciences, January 6–9, 2003.

24. Claire Honeybourne, Sarah Sutton, and Linda Ward, "Knowledge in the Palm of Your Hands: PDAs in the Clinical Setting," *Health Information Library Journal* 23 (March 2006): 51–59.

25. Wireless Internet Institute, "Wireless Technology Offers Low-Cost Internet Access to Underserved Areas," July 21, 2004.

26. Darrell M. West, *The Rise and Fall of the Media Establishment* (Boston: Bedford/St. Martin's Press, 2001), p. 28.

27. Deloitte Center for Health Solutions, "ICD-10: Turning Regulatory Compliance into Strategic Advantage," May 2008 (http://whitepapers.zdnet.com/abstract.aspx?docid=346753 [January 28, 2009]).

28. "All-Digital Hospital Opens in Ohio with McKesson Healthcare IT Systems," *Advance for Nurses* (http://nursing.advanceweb.com/editorial/content/Editorial.aspx?CC=105455 [January 28, 2009]).

29. "Cerner Demonstrates the Hospital Room of the Not-So-Distant Future," *Business Wire,* February 22, 2007 (http://findarticles.com/p/articles/mi_m0EIN/is_2007_Feb_22/ai_n27157091/pg_1?tag=artBody;col1 [January 28, 2009]).

30. John Glaser, *The Strategic Application of Information Technology in Health Care Organizations* (San Francisco: Jossey-Bass, 2002).

31. H. Hughes Evans, "High Tech vs. 'High Touch': The Impact of Medical Technology on Patient Care," in *Sociomedical Perspectives on Patient Care,* edited by J. M. Clair and R. M. Allman (University Press of Kentucky, 1993), pp. 83–95.

32. Jay Shen, "Health Information Technology: Will It Make Higher Quality and More Efficient Healthcare Delivery Possible?" *International Journal of Public Policy* 2, no. 3/4 (2007): 281–98.

33. Samuel Wang and others, "A Cost-Benefit Analysis of Electronic Medical Records in Primary Care," *American Journal of Medicine* 114, no. 5 (April 1, 2003): 397–403.

34. Robert Miller and Ida Sim, "Physicians' Use of Electronic Medical Records," *Health Affairs* 23, no. 2 (March-April, 2004): 116–26.

35. Richard Baron and others, "Electronic Health Records: Just around the Corner? Or Over the Cliff?" *Annals of Internal Medicine* 143, no. 3 (August 2, 2005): 222–26.

36. Anne-Marie Audet and others, "Information Technologies: When Will They Make It into Physicians' Black Bags?" *Medscape General Medicine* 6, no. 4 (2004): 2.

37. Jeff Goldsmith, *Digital Medicine: Implications for Healthcare Leaders* (Chicago: Health Administration Press, 2003).

38. Mark Frisse, "State and Community-Based Efforts to Foster Interoperability," *Health Affairs* 24, no. 5 (September-October 2005): 1190–96.

39. Jeff Goldsmith, David Blumenthal, and Wes Rishel, "Federal Health Information Policy: A Case of Arrested Development," *Health Affairs* 22, no. 4 (July-August 2003): 44–55.

40. "Online Health Records Urged," *Providence Journal,* October 30, 2007, p. A4.

41. Steve Ohr, "Doctors Balk at Electronic Records," *Providence Journal,* June 22, 2008, p. F4.

42. Milt Freudenheim, "A Model for Health Care That Pays for Quality," *New York Times,* November 7, 2007, p. C3.

43. J. D. Kleinke, "Dot-Gov: Market Failure and the Creation of a National Health Information Technology System," *Health Affairs* 24, no. 5 (September-October 2005): 1246–62.

44. See www.HealthVault.com.

45. Steve Lohr, "Microsoft Offers System to Track Health Records," *New York Times,* October 5, 2007, p. C3.

46. Ibid.

47. Jay Greene, "Microsoft Wants Your Health Records," *Business Week,* October 15, 2007, pp. 44–46.

48. Steve Lohr, "Safeguards Sought on Web Health Data," *New York Times,* April 17, 2008, p. C9.

49. Gordon Brown, Tamara Stone, and Timothy Patrick, *Strategic Management of Information Systems in Healthcare* (Chicago: Health Administration Press, 2005).

50. National Research Council, *For the Record: Protecting Electronic Health Information* (Washington: National Academies Press, 1997).

51. Linda Moody, "E-Health Web Portals," *Holistic Nursing Practice* 19, no. 4 (July-August 2005): 156–60.

52. Scott Gottlieb, "U.S. Doctors Want to be Paid for E-Mail Communication with Patients," *BMJ* 328 (May 15, 2004): 1155.

53. John Stone, "Communication between Physicians and Patients in the Era of E-Medicine," *New England Journal of Medicine* 356 (June 14, 2007): 2451–54.

54. Anderson, "Consumers of E-Health."

55. Skinner, Biscope, and Poland, "Quality of Internet Access."

56. Newt Gingrich with Dana Pavey and Anne Woodbury, *Saving Lives and Saving Money: Transforming Health and Healthcare* (Washington: Alexis de Tocqueville Institution, 2003); "American Health Choices Plan," September 17, 2007 (www.HillaryClinton.com); Patrick Healy and Robin Toner, "Wary of Past, Clinton Unveils A Health Plan," *New York Times,* September 18, 2007, p. A1; Perry Bacon Jr. and Anne Kornblut, "Clinton Presents Plan for Universal Coverage," *Washington Post,* September 18, 2007, p. A1; and "Barack Obama's Plan for a Healthy America" (www.BarackObama.com [May 29, 2008]).

Index